Guide to the Comatose Patient

EXPERT ADVICE
FOR FAMILIES AND CAREGIVERS

EELCO F.M. WIJDICKS

M.D., Ph.D., FACP, FNCS | Neurocritical Care, Mayo Clinic

MAYO CLINIC PRESS

MAYO CLINIC PRESS
200 First St. SW
Rochester, MN 55905
MCPress.MayoClinic.org

The information in this book is true and complete to the best of our knowledge. This book is intended as an informative guide for those wishing to learn more about health issues. It is not intended to replace, countermand or conflict with advice given to you by your own physician. The ultimate decision concerning your care should be made between you and your doctor.

Information in this book is offered with no guarantees. The author and publisher disclaim all liability in connection with use of this publication. The views expressed are the author's personal views and do not necessarily reflect the policies or position of Mayo Clinic.

To stay informed about Mayo Clinic Press, please subscribe to our free e-newsletter at MCPress.MayoClinic.org or follow us on social media.

For bulk sales to employers, member groups and health-related companies, contact Mayo Clinic at SpecialSalesMayoBooks@mayo.edu.

ISBN 978-1-893005-81-5
Library of Congress Control Number: 2021950115

Printed in the United States of America

Proceeds from the sale of Mayo Clinic Press books benefit medical education and research at Mayo Clinic.

Acknowledgments and dedication

My thanks to Mayo Clinic Press and many others who made the experience of writing this book so rewarding. I thank editors Judith Orvos and Karen Wallevand for their support in bringing the book to fruition. My deepest thanks to Lea Dacy for helping make the text more colloquial and lyrically descriptive. I am also grateful to the Mayo Clinic illustrators and data visualization specialists who assisted in this project, particularly Paul Honermann and Seth Lambert, and to production designer Amanda Knapp.

This book was written during the COVID-19 pandemic — one of the worst times in intensive care medicine. To treat severe COVID-19 and control increased respiratory drive and agitation associated with respiratory distress, many people on a ventilator are receiving very high doses of sedation, causing them to become comatose. Critically ill patients facing a lengthy awakening and recovery have become quintessential symbols of the severity of the pandemic.

Every day at work, I see patient families who are struggling and distressed but also resilient, tough, relieved and thankful. I also see devoted health care providers who guide families through very traumatic situations. This book is, therefore, dedicated to all affected by coma and the health care professionals caring for coma patients and their families. I hope this guide provides deeper understanding and, thus, solace for families as they handle an often unexpected and unfamiliar situation.

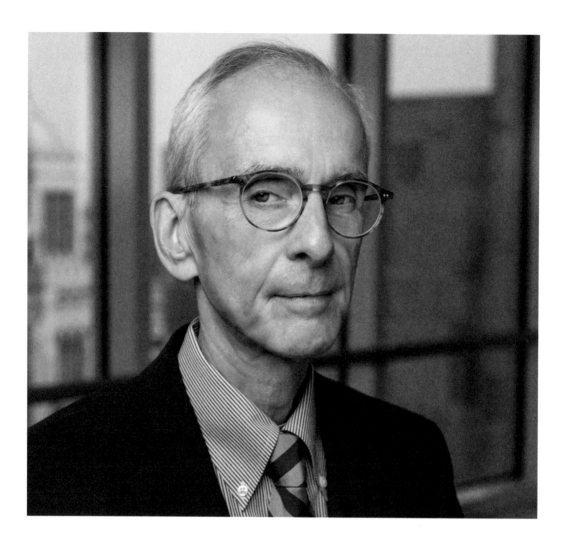

Eelco F.M. Wijdicks, M.D., Ph.D., is a neurointensivist at Mayo Clinic, Rochester, Minn., and professor of neurology at Mayo Clinic College of Medicine and Science. He established the specialty of neurocritical care at Mayo Clinic and is an attending neurointensivist in the Neurosciences Intensive Care Unit at Mayo Clinic Hospital — Rochester, Saint Marys Campus. Dr. Wijdicks is the founding editor of the journal *Neurocritical Care*, the official journal of the Neurocritical Care Society, of which he is an honorary member.

Dr. Wijdicks has published more than 1,000 research papers, practice guidelines, topic reviews, book chapters and editorials. He has authored, co-authored and edited 25 books on neurocritical care. He also created the FOUR Score coma scale to help assess the level of patient unconsciousness.

Dr. Wijdicks lives with his wife Barbara-Jane in Rochester, Minn., and Bonita Springs, Fla.

Contents

Preface

Comatose? How did that happen? Does he need brain surgery? Will he awaken? What will I notice? Will she be the same? Should I be here all the time? How long does it take for him to wake up? You say she'll wake up disabled, but I am sure she does not want to end up in a nursing home. I know what you mean by "no recovery," but can we wait a few more weeks to find out how things go? Is there nothing else you can do? I've heard so many good things about music therapy, acupuncture, hyperbaric treatment and stem cells.

I've heard these questions and statements many times. Families are understandably bewildered about what they should do and how to respond to an acute situation such as coma. All was well when the day started, but then something terrible happened. Families must now face a

new reality. Medical staff will try to explain what's happening, but the situation is complicated, and there's a lot that families may grapple with.

When the world suddenly stops, it's very difficult for outsiders to imagine what it's like. It seems unreal. Often, families need help to make sense of what is happening and what to do. This book is for families of loved ones in coma. It aims to provide answers and insight for family members faced with this hardship.

Guide to the Comatose Patient offers advice on managing uncertainties while waiting for recovery. My approach is a realistic and honest engagement with families. I share advice on how to deal with what often feels like a roller coaster ride when a loved one is hospitalized and comatose. I fully recognize that the interaction between health care staff and families is just as important to recovery and healing as is the care that a comatose individual is receiving.

Neurointensivists encounter comatose patients on a daily basis. On any given day, hospital intensive care units (ICUs) house several patients who are unconscious. Some patients in ICUs are in what's called a medically induced coma, in which anesthetic medications are used. This is often done to calm the patient and to allow a ventilator to work properly. But coma may occur for other reasons, such as drug or alcohol intoxication or traumatic brain injury. Coma also may follow resuscitation after a heart attack or another circulatory or cardiac event.

These events raise many questions: What is coma? What's a vegetative state? Will my loved one recover? Will my loved one be disabled? What does brain death mean? The list goes on. In this book, I try to answer these questions.

The human brain is a stupendous structure that can endure a lot. But brain injury can and does happen, causing various states of unconsciousness. Being comatose is often viewed as being asleep. However, unlike sleep, individuals in deep coma don't open their eyes when their names are called or wake up when they're gently shaken.

And even if a person's eyes are open, it doesn't mean consciousness. Coma can transition to the feared (though exceedingly rare) vegetative state, in which an individual has sleep cycles with periods of "sleep" and periods of being "awake" when the eyes are open. Being in a vegetative state means an individual's vegetative (automatic) functions remain, and the person continues to breathe when the ventilator is stopped and can maintain sufficient blood pressure. But the person isn't aware of surroundings, doesn't recognize family members, has a blank stare, and needs full nursing care.

Individuals in a vegetative state may remain that way for months, years, or even permanently. Their eyes may wander and remain open most of the day. This is why a vegetative state is sometimes referred to as "eyes-open coma." However, the person doesn't see, hear, feel, sense discomfort, or experience hunger or thirst. Patients in a vegetative state float in limbo between life and death.

Brain death is different. When physicians say a patient has become brain-dead, it means we see no reflexes or movement, and breathing can only happen with assistance. Blood pressure is low and can only be maintained with continuous drug infusions. Body temperature declines due to loss of temperature regulation.

These three neurologic conditions — coma, vegetative state and brain death — are not the same. Coma will often improve. Vegetative state may improve but most often it doesn't, and generally not without major consequences. Brain death is permanent, and because intensive and hard-to-maintain care is required to support the body's major organ systems, we clinically accept it as death.

When a person arrives at the hospital in a comatose state, our major concern is to avoid depriving that individual of a good outcome, if such a possibility exists. Many physicians will (and should) do all they can to allow the person the chance to improve. These measures may include surgery, medications to control swelling, and other interventions to allow the damaged brain to heal and to prevent complications, such as infections or muscle contracture.

Unfortunately, despite aggressive measures, there may be only minimal improvement or no improvement at all. When the news isn't good, questions arise about how far to go in trying to elicit a positive response and when to transition from aggressive care to comfort care.

This is a very difficult situation for family members, but families are usually in the best position to know what their loved ones would have wanted. Some families find it difficult to live with the potential consequences of a "wrong" decision, and they continue care even if improvement is highly unlikely. They rationalize that continuing care causes no harm. (Actually, it can cause harm, because treating complications often leads to more-serious complications.)

Generally, families make decisions while trying to imagine how their loved ones would respond to living with a specific, severe disability. An advance directive may help, but not always because the language in advance directives can be difficult to interpret. "If I become terminally ill, I do not want any heroic measures" is a

common phrase in advance directives. But these generic statements often confuse families. What did the individual mean by "heroic measures"?

In the past, physicians caring for comatose patients often wouldn't communicate much with families. This has changed drastically in many, though not all, countries in the world, and health care providers make themselves available to communicate with family members as much as possible.

Ongoing interaction between a physician and family is very important. Physicians must strive to be realistic and stay emotionally neutral, which isn't always easy. Physicians with an overly optimistic attitude may always see a silver lining, even when the outlook isn't good, and unnecessarily prolong care. Conversely, families may regard overly pessimistic physicians as confrontational and unpleasant, which damages the family-physician relationship.

Certainly, no families are alike, but typical trends emerge. Some families quickly understand the gravity of the situation and know that prolonged care of their loved ones doesn't make much sense. Other families think that medicine is about trying everything, no matter the cost or long-term outcome. A few put trust in a "miraculous recovery." And disagreements among family members about what their loved one would want are common.

There are books on family experiences with acute traumatic brain injury and coma, and each provides a good insight about what families go through. Many are based on faith, hope and spiritual support. This book takes a different approach. It seeks to show families the perspective of the staff caring for their loved ones. (It takes a neurologist to know what a neurologist is thinking and doing.)

I discuss what worries physicians, how we think and intervene, what we can and cannot predict, and what we know with certainty. Readers will notice the book is candid about the health care system, the role of doctors and our unease. Although I touch on my personal experiences with grieving families, this is not a personal reflection.

I attempt, to the best of my ability, to explain what we know with certainty and what we don't, and also to address misconceptions. Eventually, most patients awaken from coma, and with rehabilitation, quite a few recover reasonably well. Individuals who've been in a coma won't remember the long days in the intensive care unit and who visited them. All the tests and poking and prodding are often forgotten, and memories are far, far away. It takes weeks, if not months, for people to fully understand what has transpired and what the future holds. For individuals now living with a disability and their families, bad feelings may overshadow good ones, but often there's more to celebrate than to mourn.

Initially, the book may appear divided into two sections: hopeful (Chapters 2-4) and hopeless (Chapters 5-8). This rather equal coverage suggests that coma is a fifty-fifty proposition. While we can't (and shouldn't) forget that there are many good outcomes, poor outcomes are unfortunately more common. My goal is to convey a positive message but one grounded in reality. Facts must direct actions and predictions. There's no reason to do it any other way.

In the final chapters, I explore the physician-family relationship and explain my philosophy and how I would like physician-family interactions to work. It's a compilation of my experiences from numerous family conferences in which families offered their insights as to how medical staff can best guide and serve families. I also touch on experimental and unproven therapies, and I spend a bit of time discussing how coma is covered and portrayed in the media and its effect on families.

Each chapter begins with a conversation taken from some of my memories and mental notes. None is verbatim, but each illustrates common themes. The book includes a section on frequently asked questions that families should consider asking or that may provide answers to questions they have. Finally, at the end of the book, I've collected the major works underlying some of the statements I made.

This book has one major goal: to create an open dialogue and optimal transparency. Hopefully, it provides guidance and reassurance to those of you living through a very difficult experience. Families must keep on keeping on.

Eelco Wijdicks

What is coma?

A CONVERSATION

Physician: I'm sorry to tell you that your son has been in a terrible accident. His brain was injured, and he's been comatose since he arrived here.

Family: We didn't expect this, and we're so unprepared. It's so hard seeing him like this. Can he hear us? I thought he was squeezing my hand, but then he stiffened up. It looks like he's crying. And why is he clenching his teeth?

Physician: Your son likely isn't aware of his surroundings and what he's doing and showing us. Right now, that's a good thing. He can't feel pain from his bone fractures, and he doesn't know he's on a ventilator.

Family: What now?

Physician: First, let me explain what it means to be comatose — for him and you.

The question "What is coma?" isn't simple to answer. Unconsciousness, or coma, is a weighty subject but, so is consciousness. Human consciousness — the basis of thought and reasoning — is enduringly mysterious. So is the opposite: being unconscious or comatose, commonly referred to as being "in a coma."

Visiting someone in the hospital who's comatose can be very emotional, and family and friends often have many questions. They want to know what their loved ones are experiencing. Do their loved ones feel helpless or "locked into" their bodies? Can they sense others around them? Can they hear and understand what's being said? What will they feel, see and hear as the coma lifts? This book is my attempt to help you understand what it means to be in a coma.

The ancient Greeks used the word κῶμα (coma) for the state of deep sleep, but it doesn't describe what people who are comatose experience. The general public may talk about people being in a coma, unresponsive or "out of it" as if they mean the same things, but that's not the case. The way a comatose patient looks isn't an indication of whether he or she is responsive. The key is the patient's level of consciousness, a complex concept that I'll explain in this chapter.

CONSCIOUSNESS VS. UNCONSCIOUSNESS

Before I talk about unconsciousness, it's important to understand consciousness. Being conscious (or, in essence, thinking) is uniquely human. It's what makes us aware of who we are and what we do, and it allows us to reason. Each of us has an inner life and our own experiences on which we reflect. As human beings, we have free will. Our actions are willful when we're conscious.

No one knows where consciousness comes from. There's no specific, physical area in the brain where it resides. Consciousness is relative, too. Little is necessary for us to become less conscious of our surroundings. (If it just started raining outside, you may not have noticed because you're reading this book.)

Despite its considerable importance, human consciousness is truly one of the greatest mysteries of neuroscience and a field of renewed study, particularly by philosophers and basic neuroscientists. Over the centuries, many theories about consciousness have been discussed and discarded. We're nowhere close to having an explanation about the biologic and physical basis of the condition.

The mechanics of consciousness

The brain consists of cells and tracts. Neurons are the major working cells in the brain, and they connect with one another through multiple branches (dendrites) that extend out of them. Neurons can be grouped in a so-called nucleus. Nerve tracts are bundles of nerve fibers connecting nuclei. What we do know is that we need a certain number of connections in our brains to process, memorize, motivate and make plans.

In order to function, the networks between these connections need more than a dozen chemical substances, called neurotransmitters. Neurotransmitters are the brain's messengers. These messengers can fire up or tamp down signals coming from neurons. The discovery of neurotransmitters led to an understanding of why certain drugs affect our wakefulness and mood. But we haven't even scratched the surface in exploring the nature of consciousness — one of the ultimate questions of life.

Disease or injury doesn't usually make us lose our consciousness for good; it just lessens consciousness to some degree. When we recover, we regain thought driven by emotion (and sometimes reason). Even the most serious brain injuries don't cause people to lose their identities. For a time, however, individuals may not know where they are and may seem detached from everybody and everything.

Loss of identity after a brain injury is often the stuff of fantasy, such as what happens in Robert Ludlum's "Jason Bourne" novels or Wim Wenders' film "Paris, Texas." What the author and film director are describing is a rare condition called psychological amnesia. People diagnosed with it behave as if they don't know who they are. Zombie films often have a similar theme.

Neurologically, people are defined as being conscious if they're aware and awake. Awareness involves perception and self-monitoring. Awakeness is the opposite of sleep. Sometimes, the eyes are open and able to see, but a person isn't necessarily fully alert. For physicians, unconsciousness (coma) means that the structures in the brain that keep a person awake aren't functioning, and the person loses awareness.

The role of the brainstem

It took many years of experimental research before scientists understood which structures in the brain control awareness, how they work, and where they're located. The breakthrough came in the 1950s with the discovery that a small series of networks in the brainstem, called the ascending reticular activating system (ARAS), determines coma or wakefulness.

It seems incredible that the brainstem — a small structure underneath the brain — determines whether we open our eyes in the morning and are ready for the day, but it's true. The brainstem also directs the urge to breathe, contains cells that keep our blood pressure in check and is crucial to motor movement.

When part of the brainstem is damaged, we lose a good deal of function. But the heart, gastrointestinal system and kidneys still work because they're self-sufficient and don't require any higher-order input from the brain. If the brainstem completely ceases to function, however, all the body's essential functions are lost. I come back to this in Chapter 7.

Assessing whether a patient has impaired consciousness or is in a coma is purely a clinical judgment based on certain assessments described later in this chapter. I will explain key structures in the brain in more detail here, clarify the numerous synonyms for coma and describe the neurologic examination of patients who are comatose.

COMA VS. OTHER LEVELS OF CONSCIOUSNESS

Degrees of coma are difficult to categorize. As a result, less precise terms often are used to describe different levels of consciousness, and there's also confusion in the medical literature. Being aware of the many terms used to define unconsciousness and what those terms mean is important so that we all have the same understanding when they're used.

For years, I've been keeping a list of words I've heard people use to describe diminished consciousness. They include:
- Altered mental status
- Clouded
- Kind of out of it
- Noncommunicative
- Out of it
- Semicomatose
- Somnolent
- Sopor
- Stupor
- Unarousable
- Unresponsive

Physicians are reasonably good at recognizing the extremes of the spectrum of consciousness, which span from alertness to deep, unresponsive coma. We've also been trained to recognize conditions that mimic coma, such as locked-in syndrome

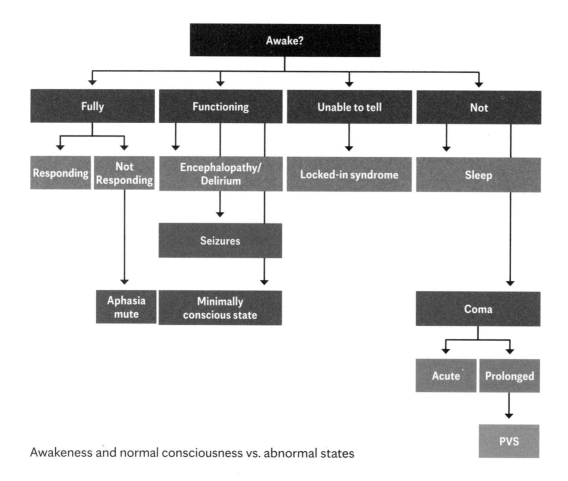

Awakeness and normal consciousness vs. abnormal states

and some psychiatric states. It's the conditions in between that pose real challenges. The spectrum of neurologic conditions is wide. Patients can present with states of consciousness ranging from being quickly responsive to stimuli, to opening their eyes only after being prodded, to remaining immobile with their eyes closed no matter what's going on around them or how much they're stimulated.

Establishing simple categories for states of awareness is often best for effective communication between family members and members of the patient's health care team. The first thing that a physician will determine when asked to see a patient who's inattentive is whether the person is awake. A range of possible diagnoses then flows from there.

The figure on the opposite page displays the normal and abnormal states of consciousness physicians encounter in patients who are hospitalized. When we see a patient who's staring quietly and inattentive, the person's condition may be hard to identify. These individuals are encephalopathic (translated as "brain disease"), which basically tells us very little. Some of them may be in delirium (delirious). Delirium includes several disturbed elements, including language, perception, orientation, mood and sleep. Traditionally, delirious patients are loud, agitated, accusatory, paranoid and offensive. Some of my medical colleagues say they've seen patients who are very quiet while hallucinating and delirious, but I'm not so sure about that. The delirium I typically see is restlessness

with sweating, rapid heart rate and wide pupils. There's a tendency to just call this acute brain failure, but vague terms have little medical value.

An individual's level of consciousness usually falls into one of five categories: alert, delirious, drowsy, stuporous or comatose:

- *Alert* patients are observant and may say hello. They are fully attentive, complete tasks promptly when asked, actively ask questions and are engaged and "with it."
- *Delirious* patients, as just described, are in a deeply disturbed state characterized by restlessness and incoherence.
- Patients who are *drowsy* can be awakened and will stay awake when engaged in conversation. They have a reduced attention span and may drift off during a conversation. Their memory is markedly impaired.
- The term *stupor* describes a condition in which the eyes remain closed if the person is lightly prodded but open in response to something painful. The individual will also tend to make movements as if to push away what's causing the pain. When the stimulation is absent, the patient immediately becomes unresponsive once again.
- The simplest definition for *comatose* is an unreceptive and unresponsive state. Unlike patients who are sleeping, those who are comatose don't wake up, speak, or open their eyes when someone talks loudly or pinches them. In response to stimuli, their arms and legs may react by withdrawing or as a reflex. If comatose patients move at all, the action isn't done with a purpose.

Lack of content also is an important hallmark of coma. Content refers to an awareness of what's happening in one's surroundings. An example would be knowing that a family member is at the bedside, recognizing the family member or being able to communicate in a rational, logical way.

People who've regained consciousness after being comatose often don't recall what happened while they were unconscious. For many individuals experiencing varying degrees of unconsciousness, it's like a veil descends on them, making them oblivious to their immediate surroundings (and, in the end, that might be a good thing). In coma, the door closes fully.

Explaining locked-in syndrome

Patients experiencing locked-in syndrome, which is very uncommon, may appear to be comatose, but they're not. Their eyes are open and the eyes blink and move vertically, but they make no other movements. These individuals are more or less awake but unable to show it. It's as if there's a major barrier they cannot overcome and they're boxed in.

Locked-in patients can feel, hear and see, but their sight is blurred by double vision because their eyes don't line up. Locked-in syndrome can occur in patients with a new brainstem abnormality (often a stroke) that involves the front of the pons. The pons is the site of several nerve bundles that create most eye movements, facial movements such as grimacing and head movements. Patients who are locked in can move their eyes vertically because the syndrome doesn't affect the upper part of the pons, called the mesencephalon, which produces vertical eye movements. Communication is possible with locked-in individuals by asking them to move their eyes vertically or to blink.

Sometimes, locked-in syndrome is triggered by medication and temporary. When people have surgery or are intubated, before the procedure, they're given a drug that paralyzes their muscles, making it impossible for them to move. Because they're sedated, however, they're not aware of this. In rare cases, the drug paralyzes the muscles, but the sedation isn't sufficient, and the person becomes very much aware of the fact that nothing moves. This may happen because the drug cleared from the person's body more quickly than what's typical or the dosage was insufficient. Again, this truly is very uncommon.

Physicians need to be fully aware of locked-in syndrome and be able to identify it based on careful examination of a patient. Some of you may be familiar with the book *Diving Bell and Butterfly* written by the former editor of *Elle* magazine who had a stroke in the brainstem that left him exactly as I have described. He was able to blink and move his eyes up and down, and he and dictated — or, if you will, blinked — the book. It became a bestseller, raising awareness about this very uncommon condition. (At the most, the large and highly advanced practice where I work sees one or two of these patients in a year.)

I mention this condition, which is outside the scope of coma, because one takeaway from *Diving Bell and Butterfly* is the revelation that nursing staff and physicians often were unaware that the book's author overheard their conversations or that the procedures he received were painful. Initially, there was nothing the author could do to convey his discomfort. Indeed, the book describes the author's feeling of "being in a nightmare" until his condition was recognized and a speech therapist helped him communicate. The syndrome has been used in movies, TV shows and novels for similar reasons: to show this most uncomfortable state. Locked-in syndrome is obviously frightening and, indeed, even nightmarish for the individual experiencing it.

Explaining a vegetative state

Coma can be prolonged, and some patients transition to a vegetative state. Neurosurgeon Bryan Jennett, M.D., and neurologist Fred Plum, M.D., coined this term in 1972. They believed that the diagnosis could only be reliably made after six months had passed and noted that the condition was extremely rare. (In the first months, a patient's condition may fluctuate too much to allow for certainty about the diagnosis.)

The European Task Force on Disorders of Consciousness subsequently proposed the term *unresponsive wakefulness syndrome* (UWS) to replace it. In doing so, the task force deliberately avoided use of the word *unawareness* and inaccurately claimed that detailed evaluation could reveal a certain level of awareness in some patients. The term *unresponsive*, however, is problematic, simply because many patients show some level of response, albeit at the level of primitive reflexes. I think unresponsive wakefulness syndrome is a very confusing term and a tongue twister, and in my experience, family members find it confusing as well.

Patients in a vegetative state open their eyes and have moments of "sleep" and "wakefulness." Their brains don't function, but from the outside, they appear conscious. These individuals are eventually able to breathe on their own. With adequate nutritional support and meticulous nursing care, many live for years and even decades. Diagnosing a vegetative state is very difficult, even for the most senior physicians. To be certain of the condition, physicians must examine an individual repeatedly over time.

Brain scans of individuals in vegetative states typically show devastating damage. In extreme cases, large parts of the brain have liquefied or calcified, confirming beyond a doubt that the individual will always need intensive medical and nursing care, as described in Chapter 2.

Only a handful of people in vegetative states surprise us by becoming more aware of their surroundings and transitioning to what we now know as a minimally conscious state. These individuals are shells of their former selves and totally dependent on 24-hour care. At times, however, they look about, make sounds, and may even say a word.

Minimally conscious patients are still very severely disabled, although some can be cared for at home. Computerized tomography (CT) scans of these individuals' brains show that their brains are shrunken and have very significant abnormalities, and many parts of the brain are out of action. (CT scans are X-rays that produce cross-sectional images of the body.)

Explaining brain death

Brain death is a state beyond coma. The term *brain death* refers to a medical state in which the automatic systems fail and the brainstem loses all its function. The hallmarks of brain death that physicians look for in a comatose patient who's experienced a known, irreversible, major structural injury to the brain are lack of brainstem function — no responses, no grimacing, no coughing, no eye movements, no limb movements, no reflexes and no breathing.

Essentially, physicians detect no signs of life. Machines and infusions are keeping the body warm and maintaining a stable blood pressure and heart rate, with air being pumped in from a ventilator every five seconds. An examination to determine if a patient is brain dead focuses on testing several brainstem reflexes and the circuitry that goes through the structures of the brainstem — the mesencephalon, pons and medulla oblongata.

If no reflexes are found, the patient is unable to breathe and medical staff has ruled out all other conditions, the person has legally died. Only then can the family consider organ donation. (More details about organ donation can be found in Chapter 7.) To neurologists and internists, a body with organs that are being artificially preserved and a nonfunctioning brain that will later liquefy is no longer a living human being.

Issues with terminology

In summary, there are a number of terms that physicians use daily as part of their medical vocabulary to describe states related to coma. Not all of them are clearly defined with specific diagnostic criteria, but we need a medical language beyond the common (but disappearing) Latinized Greek. Neurologists generally remain wary of many of these terms because they're vague and their use can mask serious evolving diseases. For now, they're labels, and most attempts to rename states of unconsciousness have led to even more ambiguity.

A final issue with terminology that bothers me is the use of metaphors for prolonged coma. Unfortunately, terms such as vegetable, plant or zombie are thrown around in nonmedical publications. Besides being deeply offensive, they're absurd. Out of respect for patients, they should never be used. I hesitated to mention them, but I continue to hear them to my dismay. I suggest using the term *prolonged coma* instead.

Patients in a prolonged comatose state deserve our care and respect. For many people, keeping a loved one in such a state indefinitely is unthinkable; for others, they feel there's still a trace of hope that their loved ones can improve, and, within reason, they want to hang on to this hope — at least for a time.

HOW DOES COMA OCCUR?

Electrical circuits are a good metaphor when it comes to explaining coma. Arguably, the most important discovery in medicine was the switch from the disproven theory of fluids — called spirits — that supposedly flowed through the nerves to sharpen the brain and muscle function, to objective, hard proof that electricity drives nerve signals.

Electricity — a physical phenomenon with no apparent connection to living systems — suddenly became fundamental to neuroscience, while animal spirits and their role in human physiology became obsolete.

We now know that neurons in the brain emit electrical signals downstream, causing neurotransmitters to jump to other neurons and ignite them. So, electrical circuits aren't too far off as an analogy for explaining coma.

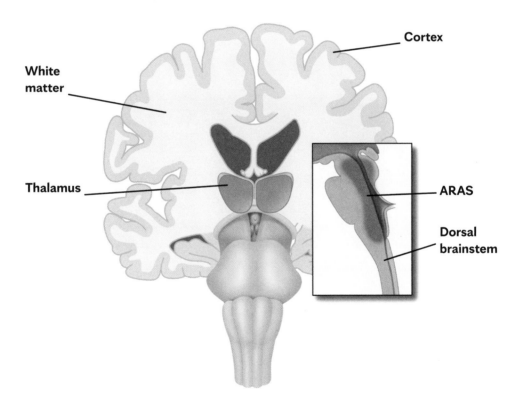

Anatomy of the main brain structures responsible for awareness

Hemisphere

Thalamus

Brainstem

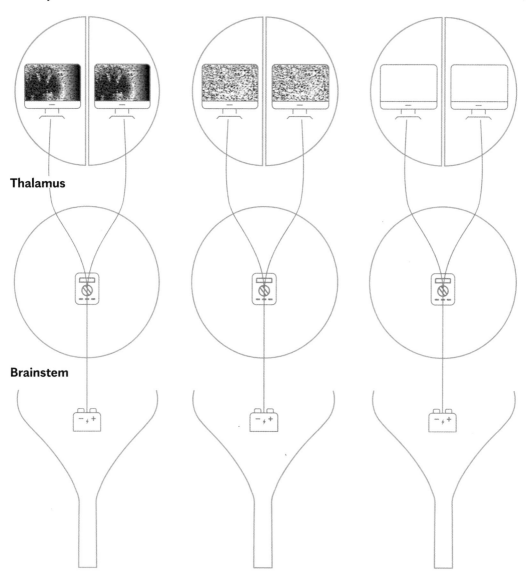

Using electrical circuits as a metaphor, the brainstem is the battery, the thalamus is the switchboard, and the other parts of the brain are represented by a computer and computer monitor. Severe delirium, stupor and a minimally conscious state are similar to a screen going in and out of focus (left). Coma and a vegetative state are like snow on the screen (middle). Brain death would be a permanent blank screen (right).

Several structures in the brain and brainstem basically "switch on the lights" in our bodies. As shown on the opposite page, the brainstem serves as the "battery." (The word for the anatomical structure is ascending reticular formation, which is a network of brain cells that produce signal-inducing chemicals throughout the brain.)

The brainstem feeds a switchboard deep in the brain, in a structure called the thalamus (see the opposite page). Parts of the thalamus can turn off and on. If a switch becomes loose and malfunctions, a person goes in and out of consciousness. There are multiple connections between the switchboard and the surface of the brain, known as the cortex. Thinking is controlled by the cortex, and in humans, this part of the brain is well developed. It provides us with a sense of time and speech, and some areas of the cortex (the limbic system) are key to emotions and memory storage.

If any of the electrical structures in the brainstem stop functioning, the overall information-processing "computers" in the brain will not continue to work. Picture the brain as a malfunctioning system in which the separate components are no longer connected. Trauma from an injury "cuts the wires" by severing nerve tracts. The same thing can happen if a stroke blocks blood flow to a part of the brain, which then dies.

Now let's expand our electrical circuit analogy to the interior workings of a television or computer monitor to explain conditions of abnormal consciousness.

Stupor and a minimally conscious state are similar to a screen going in and out of focus. A vegetative state is snow on the screen, and if signals are reaching the patient's brain, they're nothing meaningful. Coma is a blank screen, but the system can reboot. Brain death is a blank screen as well, but the system cannot be rebooted. And you cannot hook up a new screen because there's only one model; we are unique individuals.

Awakening and recovery

Many comas result from major physical injury to the brain, often from a traumatic accident. Taking an overdose of prescribed medication, using illicit drugs or having severely abnormal blood values can lead to a coma. In those cases, all the brain's structures are affected, not just one or two. Think of it as a power loss or sudden power surge.

High doses of medication can cause people to be unaware of their surroundings. This is basically the same as what happens when a person receives anesthesia before surgery. It also occurs when medication is deliberately given to someone with no or minimal brain injury to produce a drug-induced coma. In these situations, patients wake up nicely when the medication is discontinued. Sometimes, high doses of medication are given to comatose patients to facilitate placement of a tube for mechanical ventilation. This allows the ventilator to work properly and keeps the patient from "bucking" the ventilator or thrashing about and causing self-harm.

It's important to understand that when someone is comatose — whether from an injury, drug intoxication, a suicide attempt or a stroke — the degree of the injury determines the chance of awakening. Fortunately, most patients who are comatose for several days eventually awaken. The issue is whether the person will be the same and if not, if the apparent damage is permanent. Only a small percentage of people in a coma — estimates are less than 5% — remain that way for a prolonged period. And an even smaller percentage never awaken.

There often is a light at the end of the tunnel for many of the patients we see. We look for signs of improvement, such as not just opening their eyes but fixating, tracking and looking around, and occasionally trying to mouth words. Chapter 4 provides more detail on awakening and recovery.

EXAMINING A COMATOSE PATIENT

Coma changes many things about an individual — often all at once. Everyone caring for that individual must be prepared to deal with a potentially life-threatening situation. This is because comatose patients don't have normal reflexes. They can't protect their airways, allowing secretions to pool in the back of their throats. They also don't breathe sufficiently or deeply enough. Lapsing into a deeper coma relaxes the airway muscles even further, causing collapse and a dangerous lack of oxygen and eventually a buildup of carbon dioxide. This is the most common reason that

comatose patients are placed on mechanical ventilators.

A comatose patient's heart rhythm also may change suddenly, and blood pressure may drop if the heart doesn't pump regularly and forcefully enough. The individual's heart may stop, and cardio-pulmonary resuscitation (CPR) may be required to restart it. Neurologists and neurointensivists often see patients in a coma from a serious brain injury who are already on some sort of life support, such as a ventilator.

Patients experiencing cardiac arrest mostly have a cardiac problem. In a few cases, the cause of cardiac arrest isn't cardiac but neurological (a hemorrhage in the brain or brainstem, for example). Emergency physicians may discover additional neurologic findings on their examinations, prompting a CT scan of the brain to help determine a cause.

Personally, I don't think it's useful to perform a neurologic exam on a patient who isn't yet medically stable. For the examination to be useful, an individual must have a normal blood pressure, a stable heartbeat, ventilation supported by a breathing machine or sufficient oxygen, and reasonably normal laboratory values. All of these are essential to ensure a reliable neurologic examination.

Examination of an unresponsive patient with a very low blood pressure, low oxygen readings and ongoing bleeding that requires massive blood transfusion yields little useful information. In fact, I've seen many patients in this desperate condition who later perk up after their vital signs return to normal values.

What I'm looking for

Once I know that a patient is stable and I can be relatively certain that no drugs are lingering in the individual's system that could continue to depress brain function, I begin a neurologic examination. A systematic evaluation begins with a test for response to a stimulus.

Many people interpret a comatose patient's closed eyes as a lack of response and open eyes, conversely, as an indication that the person can communicate. However, even deeply comatose patients may briefly open their eyes spontaneously, but not blink. All patients in a prolonged coma will eventually open their eyes, but it may mean little. On the other hand, alert patients may be unable to open their eyes voluntarily due to swelling or bruising of the eyelids or an inability to perform this purposeful action after a major stroke.

Therefore, opening or closing of the eyes by itself isn't a significant indicator of whether a comatose patient has normal or abnormal consciousness. Fixating on objects (following objects spontaneously), looking around to see what's happening in the room, and following the examiner's finger movement when asked (known as tracking) are far more useful indicators of responsiveness.

When I examine a comatose patient, I look specifically for brain abnormalities that can cause coma. As noted earlier, they may be isolated in a single part of the brain or involve multiple areas. Identifying the affected location(s) in the brain is the quickest way to zero in on the area of damage and the probable cause of the patient's condition.

Health care providers often use scales to evaluate patients, and the most popular one in neurology is the Glasgow Coma Scale. Physicians use it to assess whether patients open their eyes; what motor responses they have; whether they can follow commands; whether they have reflexes; and whether they talk clearly, mumble or are confused. The scale is fairly simple, provides uniform ratings and is very helpful to health care providers who aren't neurologists. And it's certainly better than the vague terms mentioned previously. However, the information that scales provide is nowhere near what can be learned with a complete neurologic examination. An examination is far more complex and cannot be reduced to simple assessments.

Motor responses

My neurologic examinations usually begin with a test of how the patient responds to stimuli or a loud voice. Yelling at a patient may cause the eyes to open, and I then ask the person to follow a command. First, I address the patient gently and then more loudly, and then I shake the individual. Eventually, I apply a stimulus that would cause pain in a fully conscious person. It's important for family members who may be present to know that in patients with markedly low levels of consciousness, pain is expressed much differently than it is in conscious individuals. A grimace in a comatose patient may not be the same as one in someone who's fully alert.

A painful stimulus is necessary and only applied if a patient is in a deep coma. I do not apply it to patients who display episodes of consciousness. Neurologists are fully aware that we can do more harm than good by inducing unnecessary pain. We also know that it can be traumatic for a family member to watch as a physician approaches their seemingly unresponsive loved one and compresses the nail bed with a metal object to evoke a reaction.

Along with checking the patient's reaction to pain, I check several other reflexes. I grade motor responses as "following a simple command" to "localization," meaning that the patient notices a pinch, usually by moving an arm toward it. Nurses may call this action purposeful; we call it localization. When a patient lapses into a deeper level of coma, localization disappears.

Usually, I apply an unpleasant stimulus at the nail bed, which may cause the patient to quickly flinch and withdraw. It also may yield a primitive response in which the patient more gradually bends an arm and wrist. The worst sign is when patients stretch out their arms and legs when a stimulus is administered. This is known as extensor posturing and indicates a major brainstem abnormality, often a sign of one of the deepest levels of coma and permanent injury.

For family members in the room, these tests are hard to watch, and family may not completely understand why I'm doing them. Pressing nail beds with blunt instruments is necessary to get a good sense of how the patient responds — whether slowly or quickly, and whether the response is only triggered by applying increasingly forceful stimuli. It's also a good indicator of the depth of coma and a baseline for monitoring the patient's progress.

Grimacing may falsely suggest discomfort or even pain. Tears running down the cheek may falsely suggest crying. The body stiffening when pinched may falsely suggest the patient is fending off the examiner. These spasms are primitive responses that are innate in all of us, but they're usually suppressed by a normally functioning brain. When the brain is injured, these reflexes reappear. The stiffening response eventually may improve to bending the elbow or trying to touch other parts of the body. An example is when a patient knows where I'm pinching or can find catheters and tubes and attempts to remove them.

The next step, as patients improve, is to ask them to squeeze my fingers, to give a thumbs-up or peace sign, or to make a fist — and ask if they can perform these actions sequentially, which is even better. Physicians have grouped these responses into the following categories: localizing, flexion or withdrawal, extensor responses, and no response.

We always look for those signs and changes from one motor response to another on our daily rounds. Change can be meaningful — for example, from withdrawing to moving an arm up to the face in localizing — or not meaningful — a primitive reflex movement replaced by another primitive reflex movement.

Comatose patients may exhibit specific actions just for a brief period. Often, they do it while their families are at the bedside but not when a member of the health care team is there. We always trust the observations of family members and continue to watch for the actions they notice, particularly when the changes are major, such as progressing from a reflex response to being able to follow some instructions.

Brainstem reflexes

After checking a patient's motor responses, I assess brainstem reflexes. I'm evaluating the size of the pupils and how they respond to light directed into the eyes. The normal response to light focused on an eye is contraction and narrowing of the pupil. Lack of that response is an important indicator of a significant brain injury, either compression of the nerves that contract the pupil or an injury in the center of the brainstem, where the nerves originate.

Among individuals who are comatose, asymmetry of the pupils is common. One pupil may be slightly larger than the other or the pupils may be of very different sizes. A wide pupil — usually measured as 6 to 7 millimeters — indicates a significant injury to the brainstem, often from a

large mass in the brain that shifts the brainstem.

I also find it useful to assess the corneal reflex because its function tracks through the brainstem. Using a piece of cotton or a squirt of water, I stimulate the cornea, which typically results in closing of the eyelid. (The absence of both pupillary and corneal reflexes generally suggests a difficult situation involving injury of several parts of the brainstem.)

I then proceed to examination of the lower parts of the brainstem. In particular, I look at how the patient responds to the suctioning of secretions from the throat and mouth, which can elicit a cough or the presence (or absence) of grimacing with any stimulus.

I then look for the presence of a breathing drive. Can the patient breathe independently, or is the ventilator providing all the breaths? One way to find this out is to switch the ventilator to a mode that allows a patient to breathe independently (if able) or to briefly disconnect the ventilator and see if the patient breathes on his or her own. There are many situations in which medication or abnormal bloodwork values make it impossible for a patient to breathe independently, and physicians are well aware of them.

All of the tests I've described are necessary to assess the depth of coma. As you can imagine, absence of all these reflexes in a patient with a significant injury on a CT scan does not bode well for recovery and may even indicate that recovery is impossible. We use the words *brain death* if all reflexes are absent and the patient isn't breathing independently and needs blood pressure support with intravenous drugs.

Conditions mimicking coma

I should point out that unresponsiveness is seen in some patients who've had surgery to the frontal lobe of the brain and the hypothalamus. Their eyes are open, but they don't move. They may be breathing on their own and have all other brain reflexes. Stimulating these patients might lead to localization, but they don't follow commands or speak. This condition is called abulia and can mimic coma.

Also, unresponsiveness in patients who have all other reflexes may indicate aphasia, which is inability to speak aside from making sounds.

Unfortunately, bystanders often interpret unresponsiveness in patients as unconsciousness. However, a variety of situations can cause acute muteness, which is different from coma or a diminished level of consciousness.

It's also important to recognize the signs indicating that a patient is coming out of a seizure. Bystanders often witness only the end of a seizure and not the full episode, with twitching and contraction. So they see someone who's somewhat agitated or simply unwilling to cooperate. Individuals emerging from a seizure have an expressionless stare, fluttering eye movements and twitching in the fingers. And they may not respond when spoken

to. That's because they may still be having an active seizure even if large parts of their bodies aren't convulsing. This is known as nonconvulsive status epilepticus, and an electroencephalogram (EEG) often is very helpful in making the diagnosis.

When examining a comatose patient, I typically look for the major causes of coma and unresponsiveness. If something stands out and points towards a certain diagnosis, I spend a little more time on the symptoms we typically see with that diagnosis and discard or accept findings as we go along. The most challenging situation is a CT scan that shows no abnormalities in a patient who is deeply comatose. Often, this is related to a drug overdose or illicit drug use. Full laboratory testing and toxicology screening are necessary, as discussed in Chapter 2.

PROLONGED COMA

Coma is usually short-lived, but it may become chronic and evolve into a permanent vegetative state or, as mentioned earlier, a minimally conscious state. Physicians have a moral responsibility to consider carefully the terms they use and to understand the full implications of diagnosing a patient as being in a vegetative state, particularly if they use the adjective *permanent*.

Vegetative state

There's evidence of occasional misdiagnosis when it comes to declaring someone in a vegetative state. This error becomes apparent after a patient is transferred to a nursing home, where nurses notice that the individual has a lot more awareness than they were led to believe. The person may still be in a vegetative state but somewhat outside the usual textbook description.

The late neurosurgeon Bryan Jennett, one of the co-authors of the original paper describing vegetative state, later wrote in an editorial: *"In the 30 years since this state was first described and named it has provoked intense debate not only among clinical scientists and health professionals but also among moral philosophers and lawyers."* Jennett emphasized that: (1) cortical integrity isn't required for sudden light or sound to stimulate a startle response or an orienting reflex with the head and eyes turning briefly towards the stimulus; (2) emotional behaviors (smile or frown) show no consistent relation to an appropriate stimulus; and (3) a patient can respond to loud noise or attempts at nursing care by clenched teeth, rigid extremities, and high-pitched screaming that abate in response to soothing voices or music.

In any event, opening the eyes marks a patient's transition from coma to a vegetative state. The individual doesn't make eye contact and the empty stare is eerie. Periods of sleep and wakefulness follow, and possibly frequent yawning, teeth grinding, and to-and-fro tongue movements. A grimace or expressionless smile is common among such individuals and adds to the confusion about what they might be experiencing.

Individuals in a vegetative state may react to a visual threat, but very differently from the typical response. For example, moving a hand or fist to the face may cause blinking but not result in head-turning, flinching, grimacing, fixating, or any other conscious response. Such movements are often reflexive and never purposeful.

People in a long-standing vegetative state may scratch or rub themselves repeatedly and have restless hand movements, but they don't reach for objects or make movements that hint at a direction of reach. Routine nursing procedures may trigger an exaggerated heart rate or more-frequent breathing. When a noxious stimulus is administered to them, the only reaction may be a quickening of respiration and increased heart rate. Vegetative signs really refer to automatic functions, and that's where the name comes from.

To make a firm diagnosis of a vegetative state, a neurologist looks for additional subtle findings, such as eyes that jerk and move but don't focus on objects. Holding a large mirror in front of a patient in a vegetative state and tilting it back and forth won't cause a change in eye position, as it will in a person with some awareness. Muscle tone is often greatly increased, and reflexes may be spontaneously present, causing temporary shivers.

Minimally conscious state

Just like vegetative state, a minimally conscious state is a far-from-satisfactory term. What's minimal? Many patients have considerable awareness once stimulated or recover so well and quickly that the term almost seems to describe a temporary state. Patients in a vegetative state show no signs of being aware of their surroundings, but those who are minimally conscious display inconsistent and limited awareness. (It's as if the speed of the internet has been markedly slowed and is constantly being interrupted.)

Individuals in a minimally conscious state consistently follow people in the

FOUR SCORE COMA SCALE

In the FOUR Score scale, the letters EMBR refer to the different components that are tested and graded on a scale from 0 to 4.

THE FOUR SCORE

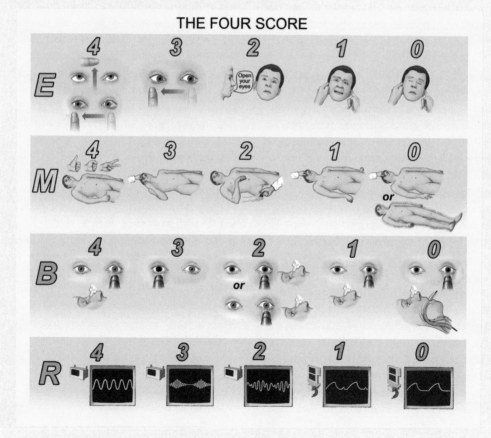

room, and they can even track a finger with their eyes. Some may even follow a very simple command or demonstrate limited purposeful behavior. However, a person in a minimally conscious state is unable to communicate reliably and consistently.

Unclear boundaries

The distinction between a vegetative state and being minimally conscious isn't always clear, and the lines may blur. It would be foolish to claim that the two conditions are always completely distinguishable.

Eye response (E)
4 = Eyelids open or opened, tracking or blinking to command
3 = Eyelids open but not tracking
2 = Eyelids closed but open to loud voice
1 = Eyelids closed but open to pain
0 = Eyelids remain closed with pain

Motor response (M)
4 = Thumbs-up, fist or peace sign
3 = Localizing to pain
2 = Flexion response to pain
1 = Extension response to pain
0 = No response to pain or generalized myoclonus status

Brainstem reflexes (B)
4 = Pupil and corneal reflexes present
3 = One pupil wide and fixed
2 = Pupil or corneal reflexes absent
1 = Pupil and corneal reflexes absent
0 = Pupil, corneal and cough reflex absent

Respiration (R)
4 = Not intubated, regular breathing pattern
3 = Not intubated, Cheyne-Stokes breathing pattern
2 = Not intubated, irregular breathing
1 = Breathes above ventilator rate
0 = Breathes at ventilator rate or apnea

Many observations and examinations are needed to confirm that a patient is in a vegetative state. Most patients in a minimally conscious state are strikingly emotionless and neither speak nor initiate spontaneous movements, but they maintain eye tracking movements, facial grimacing and blink to threat. If they hold or fondle an object, it may just be twiddling.

Patients who are more than minimally conscious or apparently improving may doodle or produce meaningless scribbles, but they cannot write with a purpose. Conventional wisdom also holds that minimally conscious patients who retain some speech have reserve sufficient to recover, and some studies suggest that the connections between the parts of their brains are better preserved than in individuals who cannot speak.

A new guideline on disorders of consciousness from the American Academy of Neurology, the American Congress of Rehabilitation Medicine, and the National Institute on Disability, Independent Living, and Rehabilitation Research, reflects concern about the reliability of the clinical diagnosis of vegetative state. This concern may be a response to some physicians who often reject a vegetative state diagnosis, preferring the patient be given a diagnosis of a minimally conscious state or better.

When this happens, it's difficult to know whether these patients have, indeed, recovered or were initially misdiagnosed. Diagnostic error rates of 40% have been cited in the medical literature, but they may be exaggerated and are dependent on who made the diagnosis and with what criteria.

The guideline suggests that about 1 in 5 patients who initially meet the criteria for a vegetative state will progress to a minimally conscious state; this also may be overblown. Factors such as who made the diagnosis and the criteria used are important. Transitions to a minimally conscious state occur primarily in younger patients with traumatic brain injuries, in whom more random outcomes are expected and who often are seen by physicians working in specialized rehabilitation centers.

Some physicians have further divided patients who are minimally conscious into those with or without language, but these subsets haven't been clearly associated with specific injuries to the brain. The diagnosis of a prolonged comatose state requires that coma exist for a year or longer before the diagnosis can be made with certainty (and, even then, with some hesitation).

AND FINALLY

I noticed over the years that the Glasgow Coma Scale didn't capture the essentials of a coma examination, and I believed that another coma scale could fill the gap. At Mayo Clinic, my colleagues and I thought this over carefully, and after considerable trial an error, we devised a new scale we call FOUR Score, an acronym for Full Outline of UnResponsiveness Score (see pages 28 and 29).

Each four-component category has a maximum grade of 4, which makes the scale easy to remember. The score is reinforced by the acronym, reminding health care staff of the most crucial parts of the examination. It works demonstrably well across disciplines, including nurses and specialists of every stripe.

The advantage of the FOUR Score is that it includes eye tracking (differentiating a vegetative state from lesser states of disordered consciousness) and blinking (excluding locked-in syndrome). When the FOUR Score is 0, it's very likely that a patient has lost all brain function, assuming that there are no other explanations for the absence of brainstem reflexes and a breathing drive. We've used the FOUR Score during an initial assessment and to monitor patient worsening.

Its reliability is equal to or higher than that of other such scales, including the Glasgow Coma Scale, and it has been validated in patients with many different disorders. Due to its proven record, the FOUR Score is an important tool in the evaluation of comatose patients in a hospital setting, and it provides neurologic findings that are crucial for grading the depth (and thus severity) of coma.

In the following chapters, I dig deeper into the causes of coma, available treatments, and other helpful approaches or measures. Recovery pathways and what to look for in patients emerging from a coma are discussed. In addition, I address considerations for compassionate end-of-life care for patients who, unfortunately, will not recover.

CHAPTER | 2

What causes coma?

A CONVERSATION

Family: We don't understand what's happening to our sister. We know she had surgery, and we were told that her CT scan was very bad and there might be brain swelling. We heard the report, but we don't know what it means. Can you help us understand all of this?

Physician: A CT scan doesn't tell the whole story. It's important to put it into perspective. Let me tell you about your sister's brain injury and what the neuro-surgeons did during surgery after she arrived at the hospital. This will help you understand what we're trying to do for her and what you can anticipate in the future.

Family: It would be good to see the scan for ourselves with you explaining it to us.

Physician: Definitely. I'll review the cause of her coma and her scans with you.

Coma may result from many medical and neurologic conditions, and its presence in the hospital may be widespread. I could easily come up with 100 causes for coma, covering all possible scenarios. Mostly, however, physicians see only a few common causes, which is why I'm going to focus narrowly on those.

The results of a neurologic examination, a computerized tomography (CT) scan of the brain or an electroencephalogram (EEG) that records electrical (brain wave) activity, and a full panel of laboratory tests often are enough to explain why someone is comatose.

Physicians get concerned when a patient is totally unresponsive but has normal vital signs, a pristine CT and normal values on laboratory tests. In those situations, our approach must be systematic and not just guesswork. In addition to a full neurologic evaluation, good medical history taking is key, relying, of course, on the accounts of others. Then, with the help of previous experience and a whole lot of common sense, we try to combine and unite the information.

For this to work, physicians have to prioritize large bits of information and determine which are most relevant. We take a hierarchical approach as we gather the strands. The challenge is to interpret the available information quickly but correctly. I described a neurologic examination in Chapter 1. Here, I'll focus on why coma occurs.

WHEN THE BRAIN IS INJURED

Before I explain brain injuries, it's important for you to understand how the brain typically functions. It's a highly active machine that needs fuel continuously, more than any other organ in the body. This fuel, in the form of sugar and its components, must always be present and can't be stockpiled for later use.

Brain cells need continuous energy to keep working, to move molecules across sheets of cell lining, and to create electrical signals using substances called neurotransmitters. When an electrical signal reaches the end of a neuron, it triggers the release of small sacs containing neurotransmitters. The body releases both stimulating (excitatory) neurotransmitters and dampening (inhibitory) neurotransmitters.

The brain is very vulnerable to injury. It can tolerate small injuries over a long period of time ("death by a thousand cuts"), but a sudden, overwhelming injury causes immediate damage and interrupts the finely tuned, synced, sublime processes that have evolved over billions of years. The brain's anatomy changes, too, with a loss of the connections and circuits needed for it to function.

The biochemistry of the demise of brain cells can be summarized in several ways. One way is to view it as a loss of control mechanisms and defenses — the drawbridge is down with the barbarians at the gate. Damage to brain cells opens the gate, allowing destructive substances to enter, which causes the machinery to malfunction and eventually grind to a halt. It's also known that once a process is set in place, a preprogrammed downfall can't be stopped. The cell literally disintegrates, and a number of chemical reactions cause protective cell layers to fail.

This cell death process, known as apoptosis, has been compared to the browning and shedding of the leaves of a tree, but sadly, there's no springlike return of new shoots. Dead cells swell, and scarred cells appear later. Alternatively, parts of the brain liquefy and later dry out and calcify. Once a neuron is lost, nothing can be done. This is an important piece of information: If a patient's coma is caused by massive destruction of the brain, the person won't recover. At best, any natural repair of the brain will likely be poor and disorganized. That's why it's important to look for the cause of a coma, the extent of the individual's injury and any other factors that play a role.

Damage to large parts of the brain from lack of blood flow and oxygen deprivation is more serious than, for example, minor trauma to the brain due to a drug overdose or intoxication. Once the drugs clear from the person's system, the coma lifts and recovery may go well. But serious or strategically placed injury to some areas of the brain — particularly the cortex, thalamus and brainstem, which are necessary to awaken us — often has major consequences.

Identifying brain injury

Advances in imaging technology have allowed us to quickly obtain good pictures of the brain. These images are essential and provide snapshots in real time of an evolving brain injury. Magnetic resonance imaging (MRI), which is now consistently used in hospitals, has markedly reduced the number of patients whose comas are unexplained. With MRI, we can see all the components of a brain injury and better understand what's going on. Before that we only had CT imaging, and some structures, such as the cortex and white matter, may appear deceptively normal on CT after an injury.

Imaging of the brain also has improved tremendously over the last decade. With functional MRI — imaging of what the brain does functionally and how it reacts to outside stimuli — we can see how the brain responds or doesn't respond and whether it can pick up outside signals. Functional MRI has been used to peek inside the brains of patients who are chronically unresponsive, and some of what we've learned is surprising. What it all means is another matter, widely open to interpretation — a fool's errand for some and, for others, a scientific revolution. (I discuss this issue in more detail in Chapter 10.)

Monitoring brain electrical activity in comatose patients by way of an EEG has some value, but its diagnostic role has never been defined (or appreciated) because brain waves are often very nonspecific. In fact, when someone has seizures, we often examine them at the bedside. If a physician isn't sure whether a patient is seizing, then an EEG can help detect specific brain activity.

In this chapter, I offer a look over the shoulders of physicians who must rapidly determine the cause of a patient's coma. The five W's plus some other factors apply here. We already know the who and when; the why, where and which follow.

THE WHY, WHERE AND WHICH

Why is a patient in a coma? Where is the injury? Which parts of his or her brain are involved? A neurologic assessment of a person who's comatose is the sum of its parts. We watch for movements, twitches and unusual positions of the eyes and limbs. We assess for responsiveness to stimuli (prods and pinches) and, most importantly, we look for signs that indicate abnormal function in either the brain hemispheres or the brainstem. Once we make these determinations, the next step is to assess the extent to which the brainstem is involved.

The brainstem plays a major role in decision-making, and abnormalities in its function provide critical information. That's why the first things physicians check are brainstem reflexes: responses of the pupils to light, blink (corneal) reflex, and eye movements provoked by moving the head. One abnormal pupil suggests a mass pressing on the oculomotor nerve that comes out of the upper brainstem. Involvement of both pupils suggests an injury to the brainstem itself.

Conversely, when brainstem reflexes are normal, we can often localize the injury to brain hemispheres. We may find either an injury (bleeding, bruising, stroke, infection) or abnormal function induced by drugs or a chemical imbalance, such as a very low blood sugar or sodium level. A CT scan or MRI scan can narrow the scope.

We use "top-down logic," meaning that we begin with what we most suspect. We try to prove our suspicions based on what we find and what we're missing. Like Captain Renault in *Casablanca*, we "round up all the usual suspects," but often we have a specific one in mind. And then we work our way through the findings, rejecting or accepting as we go along.

This stepwise practice is essential because brain scans may show one thing and the

examination something else. If the two don't agree, we have to find another cause that may be contributing to the condition. For example, we may find a clot on one side of the brain that's not putting pressure on the other side (remember from Chapter 1 that a coma involves both parts of the brain), the individual's blood glucose level may be too high or too low, sodium levels may be very low, or there may be another unexpected laboratory finding that explains what's happening.

As another example, imagine the case of someone found comatose on the street late at night. A brain scan shows a small bruise and a tiny amount of blood that's mostly outside the brain. Given that this person was near a bar, it's logical to conclude that the coma was caused by alcohol intoxication and that the bruise is likely insignificant and simply a result of the fall.

Time is of the essence in performing CT scans on comatose patients, because in most instances, the results will point to the cause of the impaired consciousness. We also clearly recognize that CT scans provide quick snapshots of the brain, and as an individual's condition evolves, more than one may be needed.

Some injuries, however, are difficult or impossible to see on regular CT scans. In those cases, MRI is a great help (and frankly, sometimes, an eye-opener) because it shows a lot more. A CT generally is most useful to quickly rule out major causes of a coma, whereas MRI reveals subtleties missed with CT scans.

Many causes

There are several causes of acute brain injury associated with a variety of known pathologic processes, such as damage from lack of blood supply, direct injury by force, or inflammation from viruses, bacteria and other pathogens. Identifying how an individual's coma developed advances the understanding of the situation. Like any other organ, the brain is vulnerable to direct injury. It may also experience indirect injury when other organs, such as the liver, heart and kidneys, fail. When that happens, the brain becomes the proverbial innocent bystander.

The accompanying chart lists causes of coma, some of which are depicted in upcoming illustrations. Rarely in medicine is the cause of a condition the same in every person. In the case of a coma, the trigger may be trauma, a shortage of oxygen, low body temperature, low blood pressure or an ongoing blood infection.

It's important that doctors recognize signs and symptoms of each of these conditions because their existence explains why one person in a coma is so badly off, while another is faring pretty well.

Persistent coma from an acute brain injury often is due to severe trauma directly to the brain. It also happens when little or no oxygen (anoxia) is getting to the brain, which may result from a drug overdose. Let's concentrate on these two common causes first. I'll then discuss other less common causes of coma.

TYPES OF ACUTE BRAIN INJURY THAT MAY CAUSE COMA

- *Vascular* — not enough blood in ischemia, too much in hemorrhage
- *Traumatic* — damage through blunt force and bruising or tearing of structures
- *Inflammatory* — infection or a reaction of the immune system
- *Obstructive* — blockage in spinal fluid circulation and enlargement of the ventricles related to blood, cancer or pus
- *Environmental* — electricity, water, ice, heat
- *Severe laboratory abnormalities* — changes in blood content, such as very low sodium or blood sugar
- *Overstimulation* — such as occurs from seizures

Direct injury

The brain and the many small blood vessels within it can't withstand much injury. Traumatic brain injury (TBI) can happen to anyone in an unguarded moment. The vast majority of these injuries are due to falls, motor vehicle accidents, sports-related injuries and assaults.

TBI can be categorized by mechanism (closed or penetrating the skull), by type of injury (inside brain tissue or external pressure) and also by its severity.

These illustrations show common causes of coma associated with brain injury.

Direct impact injury

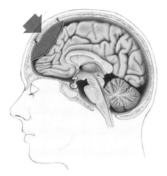

Acceleration-deceleration injury

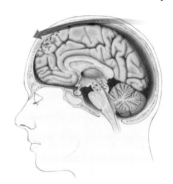

A. Direct impact from a traumatic brain injury causes blood to collect on the surface of the brain (subdural hematoma) and press on the brain, shifting brain tissue. In an acceleration-deceleration injury resulting from an abrupt stop, the brain hits surrounding hard layers of bone, causing major bruising. And the brain may swing back to the opposite side, causing more bruising. The brainstem may be bruised as well.

Ischemic stroke

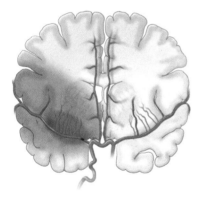

Hemorrhagic stroke

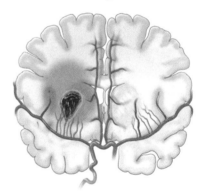

Ischemic strokes occur when arteries to the brain become narrowed or blocked, causing severely reduced flow (ischemia).

Hemorrhagic stroke occurs when a blood vessel in the brain leaks or ruptures.

B. In the case of a stroke, there's no blood flow to important parts of the brain (ischemic), or leakage from an artery is causing blood to clot (hemorrhagic).

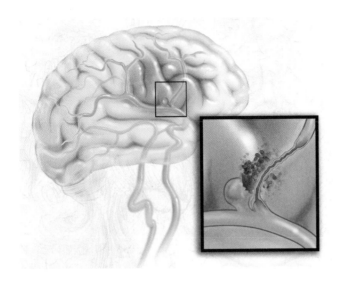

C. A subarachnoid hemorrhage results when a brain aneurysm bursts, increasing pressure inside the skull.

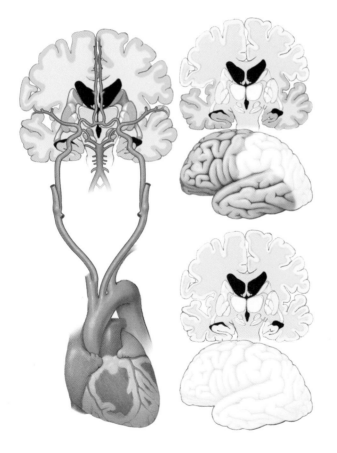

D. With cardiac arrest (no effective heart pumping), there's no blood flow to the brain's cortex. The damage is often in the most vulnerable areas of the brain (parietal occipital cortex and deeper structures) or the damage is throughout the entire cortex.

Severity of concussion relates to stretching and deformity of brain tissue from direct impact or mechanical tearing of brain tissue that leads to bleeding. Injury can also occur from tears in large arteries, which lead to a stroke.

As shown on page 38, a direct hit to the skull can produce injury at the site of impact and in other areas as the brain is thrust against the bone on the other side of the head. When evaluating a comatose patient, physicians look for skull fractures, particularly those that might cause a major dent. When present, they must be assessed immediately by a neurosurgeon to determine whether the lining of the brain has been torn. A broken bone at the base of the skull (basilar skull fracture) may be associated with vascular lacerations, particularly carotid artery trauma. Rapid acceleration or deceleration, such as a sudden car stop, can cause brain tissue to rip as it's pulled from its usual location.

In addition to the injury, there are also other insults to the brain that are just as important as the initial impact and may even be worse. Factors such as lack of oxygen and significant blood loss also can occur and happen quickly. Some studies have found that 1 in 3 patients with a severe traumatic brain injury has low blood pressure very soon after the injury. Not unexpectedly, that doubles the chances of a poor outcome or death.

Physicians who see patients with traumatic brain injuries in an emergency room (ER) immediately prioritize treatment of that condition, assuming there's no evidence of life-threatening trauma to other organs. Generally, after an individual is stabilized, we assess for increased pressure in the brain. If it's present, we may need to remove a clot.

In many ERs, as soon as a comatose individual is brought in, physicians begin monitoring brain pressure so that immediate action can be taken to reduce the pressure, if needed. A severe injury to the brain causes swelling, which increases pressure, but it may be delayed. The earlier we can get a handle on the pressure, the better. We also have come to realize that pressure may rise very quickly in people whose brains have been ravaged by penetrating injuries, and there's little we can do.

A common form of trauma to the brain after a fall is a blood clot on top of the brain — under or above the hard, outer lining known as the dura. This is also called a subdural (under) or epidural (above) hematoma. Initially, the clot may not appear to cause problems, but such an injury can lead to a severe headache and an altered state of responsiveness, resulting in a deep coma.

An individual who has a traumatic brain injury is often prepped for possible surgery if he or she has an epidural or subdural hematoma, particularly if there's also a decrease in consciousness, weakness in an arm or leg, or trouble speaking. Urgent removal of a clot by a neurosurgeon is lifesaving; however, the surgical scar can cause problems later. The area underlying the site of the clot may produce seizures because it's been injured as well. Some people who have traumatic brain injuries, especially older individuals, may never be the same.

Traumatic brain injury often is associated with a deep, unresponsive coma, and family members may arrive to find their loved one with a multitude of bruises, splints and bandages, and drains if brain surgery has been performed. To control agitation, a loved one may be heavily sedated, which can induce an even deeper coma.

It's often difficult for medical staff to get a good sense of how responsive comatose individuals are, and other data are needed to assess their conditions, including a CT scan and laboratory tests. In other words, these patients may look much worse than they really are. In the days ahead, the physician may lighten the sedation intermittently to look for responses. Family members must be prepared not to make too much of what they see, especially before they've had a chance to speak with the attending physician.

Undoubtedly, the worst trauma to the brain is what's called a penetrating injury, from a bullet or some sharp object such as a nail from a nail gun. When a sharp object passes through the brain and exits on the other side, the injury isn't survivable. When it remains on one side of the brain, there's a chance of survival. If a young person has a penetrating brain injury, the degree of the injury and results of the initial examination will determine the outcome. Coma and penetrating brain injury are truly luck of the draw and often sheer luck if someone survives with good or acceptable function and can be fully independent of others.

Too little oxygen

Oxygen is carried by a protein in blood called hemoglobin. Hemoglobin must be present in sizable quantities so that oxygen can bind to it. Limited oxygen to the brain can occur when hemoglobin binding is reduced because oxygen levels are impaired by lung disease or when oxygen competes with carbon monoxide and loses, such as what happens in carbon monoxide poisoning. The medical term for lack of oxygen is anoxia. Anoxia also occurs when hemoglobin binding is normal, but shock inhibits blood flow to the brain.

Unquestionably, a severe reduction in blood oxygen may damage the brain. Low oxygen often is associated with a marked drop in blood pressure or lack of a pulse for a brief period. Thus, the individual experiences a double hit of low oxygen and low blood pressure. Low oxygen alone is rarely a cause of brain injury. There's usually some other contributing factor that can be singled out as the main culprit.

In an individual whose injury is associated with anoxia and who remains in a coma, a CT scan may not show much. MRI is far more helpful and can show injury in areas vulnerable to low blood pressure in combination with low oxygen. Some areas of the brain are dependent on several blood vessels, each of which plays a part in the cascade of events. The areas affected are deep inside the brain and quite crucial for connections to the major command center located at the surface of the brain, known as the cortex.

Blood flow within the body is regulated by the brain. The brain supplies more blood when the pressure is too low and less when the pressure becomes too high. This is known as cerebral autoregulation, in which the brain automatically adjusts to demand. A brief reduction in blood flow or pressure results in widening of the arteries. A brief increase in blood flow or pressure produces narrowing of the arteries. Autoregulation differs among individuals. Prolonged periods of low blood pressure can be absolutely devastating for many people, but others have experienced few harmful effects.

Adequate oxygen to the brain via blood flow is critical. Here are some sobering facts. Oxygen stores are depleted within 20 seconds after the heart stops beating. Blood sugar (glucose), stored in minimal amounts, is gone minutes later. The impact on brain neurons is dire, causing a rapid lack of fuel supply and the creation of a dead core. When only a small area of the brain is affected, some reversal of this process is still possible. The compromised area surrounding the dead core (penumbra) maintains intact protective membrane pumps and high-energy metabolism, but electrical energy in the neurons stops. Restoring blood flow can reverse this state.

It's less clear if restoration is possible when there's widespread lack of blood flow during cardiac arrest or resuscitation. Even with the best techniques, resuscitation may provide only a fraction of the blood flow essential to the brain. That's because certain areas of the brain are very vulnerable, and less than 10 minutes of interrupted blood pressure and fuel supply are enough to produce cell death.

Areas of the brain most vulnerable to interrupted blood flow and oxygen depletion are the back side of the brain, where several arteries intersect (parieto-occipital region), and the cortex. The cortex is the outer surface of the brain involved in thinking, feeling and movement. The spinal cord also is vulnerable. The brain isn't just the "thinking parts," most often shown in drawings but also the brainstem.

The brainstem is the most vital part of the brain and also the last to go. That resilience is the result of an evolutionary process. Total loss of brainstem function is rare in people who are comatose, but when it happens, the brain has reached a point of no return. The brainstem is of crucial importance. The late neurologist Fred Plum, an authority on coma, wrote, *"The reader may justifiably ask: Why the brainstem? That's not where my consciousness comes from. The reason is straightforward; The brainstem holds the critical nerve centers that make brain life possible. In the brainstem lie the structures that wake us up, the nervous centers that control the pupils inside your eyes, and all of the muscles that move your eyes. In the brainstem reside the sensors that allow us to hear, as well as those that give us the capacities to sense touch, taste and a full mouth rather than an empty one. Without the brainstem we could neither chew nor swallow nor breathe ... without a brainstem I am nothing but a hopeless collection of organs, incapable of human vitality."*

Stroke

Severe (acute) stroke occurs when parts of the brain stop functioning because of lack of blood flow or due to a blood clot. Individuals are immediately alert after an acute stroke, although some of them may be stunned. Their consciousness isn't likely to be abnormal because most acute strokes occur in small sections of the brain's arteries or they involve a single part of the brain, barely affecting the structures that govern alertness and awareness.

Coma can happen after a stroke if a blood clot (embolus) develops in the main artery of the brainstem (basilar artery), destroying structures in the brainstem that govern alertness. Bleeding (hemorrhage) into the brainstem or the brain's thalamus and cortex also can cause a decline in alertness. Initial destruction of crucial brain areas is often the main cause of a coma in individuals with deep hemorrhages. A gradual decline in consciousness is more common.

In both an ischemic stroke (no blood flow) and hemorrhagic stroke (blood clot), coma generally indicates development of additional swelling due to the bleeding or dead tissue. Coma definitely can occur if someone has a stroke involving the brainstem or if the brainstem is under pressure due to swelling in the structure located under the brain (cerebellum).

Coma may also result if an aneurysm ruptures. An aneurysm is an enlargement or bulge of an artery caused by a weakening of the artery wall. Many aneurysms occur outside of or at the base of the brain. As a result, individuals who experience them typically don't lose consciousness and remain alert. However, pressure inside the brain can build enough to stop blood flow, causing the brain to stop functioning — a sort of brain arrest. Coma may also result when the fluid-filled chambers in the brain (ventricles) become blocked and enlarge, placing pressure on nearby brain structures.

At the onset of an aneurysm, it's impossible to know whether an individual's injury will be permanent. The individual may never recover, or he or she may recover after the aneurysm is repaired and increased pressure in the brain is relieved.

Hypoglycemia

Severe low blood sugar (hypoglycemia) can cause brain injury. This often is due to an overdose of insulin or a medication error. Hypoglycemic brain injury, resulting from not enough blood sugar (glucose) to fuel the brain's cells, differs biochemically from reduced blood flow. However, hypoglycemia may be accompanied by reduced blood oxygen levels and shock. This means coma may be a combination of the two conditions, an example of an interconnection between different types of injury that can result in persistent coma.

Infection

An infection of the brain's central nervous system can result in severe, rapid injury. Bacteria don't enter the brain easily because of the blood-brain barrier, a semipermeable border designed to prevent pathogens (viruses, bacteria and other microorganisms) circulating in blood from entering the brain. However, once they pass that obstacle, they multiply rapidly in the fluid compartments of the brain, including cerebrospinal fluid, and cause an inflammatory response. Initial swelling (edema) indicates that fluid can more easily pass through the blood-brain barrier. Later on, reduced flow of cerebrospinal fluid from the brain can add to the swelling.

The flow of cerebrospinal fluid may be impeded by high resistance in the small protrusions (arachnoid villi) that help move fluid from the thin second layer of the brain into the thicker outer layer. Clotting abnormalities in infected brain arteries also may play an important role. Markedly decreased cerebral blood flow due to spasm in the arteries and inflammation may be an important component.

All of these mechanisms may be operating before a patient receives the first dose of antibiotics intended to destroy the infection-causing pathogens. In addition, as the walls of bacteria cells are destroyed, they may release products that increase brain inflammation.

Acute demyelination

A less common cause of acute brain injury is acute demyelination. In this condition, a protective covering around nerve fibers (myelin) is attacked by cells that inflame or destroy it. Microscopic examination of tissue can reveal loss of myelin with preservation of nerve cells and fibers. However, if demyelination affects bundles of nerve fibers, is severe and progresses rapidly, it can produce a mass in the brain or spread diffusely throughout the white matter. As this happens, nerve impulses slow or even stop, leading to coma.

Prolonged seizure

The brain can sustain damage from overexertion, which can happen when a brain seizure lasts an hour or more. The overheating stress on brain neurons is so high that "the kettle explodes." This is far more common in patients with a flurry of seizures. If the first seizure is prolonged, or if a second seizure occurs, physicians generally prescribe anti-seizure drugs to prevent additional seizures. Recent research indicates overworked neurons can damage themselves.

Seizures result from an imbalance between brain inhibition (dampening down) and excitation (revving up). The substances formed during seizures (excitatory amino acids) also play a role in epilepsy-associated injury. During seizures, sodium and calcium enter the cells and cause them to be overly excited.

To complicate matters, each of these abnormalities can cause additional injury through brain swelling. When the brain swells, tissue is moved where it doesn't belong and may make its way into natural openings between brain compartments. That's why steps to prevent a secondary injury— not just treating the initial injury — are an important part of caring for an individual with a neurologic injury. A secondary injury can change the outlook markedly.

INITIAL EVALUATION AND TREATMENT

Individuals in a coma are generally first seen in the emergency department or in the intensive care unit (ICU). It's much less common for individuals in other areas of the hospital to deteriorate suddenly and become comatose.

In the emergency department

I would wager that the majority of neurology consultations in emergency departments among patients experiencing coma are overdose-related. Given the opioid epidemic, many emergency departments frequently treat overdoses and deal with a number of associated issues, including whether persistent coma can be reversed.

In the emergency department, the cause of a coma often quickly becomes clear following a CT scan of the brain. The scan can show traumatic brain injury, acute cerebral hemorrhage, and severe brain swelling, among other things. When a CT scan comes back normal and there are no identifiable signs suggesting injury to a specific area of the brain, intoxication is a likely cause.

In these situations, physicians often look to ethanol or atypical alcohols and heroin or other opioids (such as fentanyl and carfentanil) as potential causes. An overdose of benzodiazepines used to treat anxiety and panic attacks also can result in coma. In cases of intoxication due to drug ingestion, an individual may experience seizures.

We consider several drugs to treat the intoxication. Coma resolves quickly if an antidote to the drug that caused it is available. For example, naloxone can be sprayed into the nose to treat an opioid overdose. Often, however, intoxication is best managed with supportive care and a wait-and-see approach.

The challenge is to decide whether supportive care alone will suffice (in a very stable patient), whether the toxin should be actively removed (in a highly unstable patient), or whether the effect of the toxin should be mitigated (in an intermittently unstable patient).

Antidotes need to be carefully considered, and may not be used because of their potential side effects. Naloxone, for example, can cause aspiration from rapid arousal and lead to a major withdrawal syndrome characterized by severe agitation and, as a result, heart rhythm disturbances. Flumazenil reverses benzodiazepine intoxication, but its use can cause arousal, vomiting, aspiration and seizures in patients with certain predispositions.

In the ICU

In addition to individuals who arrive in the emergency department and are later transferred to an ICU, a neurologist may see patients in an ICU for a variety of reasons.

Failure to awaken after surgery is one reason. This is often related to the effects of medication. A neurologist will evaluate an individual's medications to see whether any changes were made recently or new medications started. Among organ transplantation patients, failure to awaken is generally sedation-related because sedation is common in very critically ill patients.

Failure to awaken may also be associated with liver injury that slows the breakdown of the drugs. It also may be related to events that happened during surgery, such as the development of low blood pressure (hypotension). Electrolyte changes, such as a severe drop in sodium, may be another potential factor.

Failure to awaken after major cardiovascular surgery may indicate a lack of blood flow to the brain during surgery (anoxic-ischemic injury), even in the absence of a clear cause such as high blood pressure or cardiac arrest. Another possibility is formation of blood clots during surgery that travel to the brain causing strokes.

Individuals who experience life-threatening abdominal or orthopedic trauma from an injury or accident often undergo immediate surgery. These individuals may be alert, and a brain CT scan prior to surgery may be normal. If they don't awaken after surgery, they may have experienced bruising of the brain from the accident or injury and now may be experiencing delayed bleeding in the brain (hematoma).

Failure to awaken may also be associated with sepsis. Sepsis is the body's extreme response to an infection. It occurs when chemicals released in the bloodstream to fight an infection trigger serious inflammation. Individuals with sepsis may not awaken after medications to sedate them are stopped. Oftentimes, a CT scan or MRI is normal, which makes the situation even more challenging.

There's no satisfactory explanation for prolonged coma after severe sepsis. Multiorgan failure is a common endpoint in patients who survive severe sepsis. Major brain dysfunction also can result.

In non-ICU areas

It's highly unusual for patients hospitalized in general medical or surgical wards to lose consciousness. Severe low blood sugar (hypoglycemia) or high blood sugar (hyperglycemia) are the most likely causes. Occasionally, too much sedation may be a factor.

In individuals with advanced cancer, seizures can occur, which may be related to spread (metastasis) of the cancer to other organs or to recent chemotherapy. Bleeding associated with metastatic cancer also can lead to coma, as can other conditions affecting the central nervous system or an immune system reaction to the tumor (paraneoplastic syndrome).

Acute respiratory failure is one more reason for coma to occur outside the ICU. Individuals who take opioid medications to manage pain, such as surgery patients or individuals hospitalized with cancer, may experience breathing that's too shallow (respiratory hypoventilation), resulting in high levels of carbon dioxide in the bloodstream.

Long-acting opioids and dermal patches are notorious for causing a sudden decline in consciousness after an individual seemed to tolerate the first dose quite well. Fortunately, too much carbon dioxide in the bloodstream (hypercapnia) is fully reversible after a short period of being on a ventilator.

Other, less common reasons for coma include the development of fat particles in the bloodstream among individuals who've had surgery to repair major fractures in the body's long bones. The condition can cause a rapid decline in consciousness. Although rare, acute coma also can occur in an individual after delivery of a healthy baby due to amniotic fluid entering the bloodstream. Stroke is one of the most common neurologic complications of pregnancy and can occur if blood pressure rises very quickly.

Looking for clues

When the cause of coma isn't obvious and an individual's CT scan is normal, physicians often turn to paramedics, family members and bystanders for help. Some of the questions we ask may seem intrusive, but the answers could be essential to understanding what led to the coma.

- *Could this be a major lack of oxygen or blood flow to the brain?* How was the person found? What did the area around him or her look like? Was he or she breathing when first responders arrived? Was there a cardiac arrest, and how long did resuscitation efforts last before the person's heartbeat and blood pressure were restored? Was there noticeable blood loss? Did the person's condition deteriorate during transport?

- *Could this be an overdose?* What pills does the person have access to? Are there needle tracks? Is the individual a habitual drug user or drinker? Has he or she made prior suicide attempts or had a psychiatric consultation? Are there problems at work? Has anyone complained about the person's drug or drinking habits? Could he or she have taken an overdose of drugs (their own or someone else's) that lowered blood sugar?

- *Could this be an infection?* Was the person taking antibiotics for an infection? Was there a rapid onset of fever and headache? The possibility of a brain infection must always be considered when someone has a rapid onset of fever and headaches, acts confused, and seems to be developing a speech impediment. A CT scan is often normal in individuals with acute infection. Cerebrospinal fluid should be examined quickly if there's a possibility of infection. Failure to recognize an infection could have major consequences. The best course of action for individuals in an infection-related coma is immediate treatment with broad-spectrum antibiotics and antiviral drugs even before receiving the results of pathogen tests.

- *Could this be low blood sugar or very high blood sodium from dehydration?* Does the person have diabetes, or could the person have undiagnosed diabetes? If the person has diabetes, has he or she had difficulty controlling blood sugar levels and was there a recent change in medication to treat it? Did the person have poor access to fluids or was he or she on water pills (diuretics)?

- *Could the coma be caused by a seizure?* Does the individual have epilepsy?
- *Could this be a clot in the basilar artery?* Is the person known to have an irregular heart rate, atrial fibrillation or another cardiac condition? Were anticoagulation medications recently discontinued? Was his or her high blood pressure poorly controlled?
- *Could this be due to extremely high blood pressure?* Extremely high blood pressure makes blood vessels leaky, and swelling occurs in the surrounding brain tissue. Did the person recently start taking transplantation anti-rejection drugs? Anti-rejection drugs are notorious for causing brain swelling due to leaking blood vessels?

Even after these questions are answered, we still may not know the cause of the coma. In these cases, an MRI (or a series of them) may be helpful if an individual doesn't improve. MRI technology has solved problems many times.

Brain imaging

When imaging tests are performed on individuals in a coma, doctors will generally discuss the results of the tests with loved ones and point out any injuries that are found or areas of concern.

CT findings

CT imaging of the brain is the quickest way to identify possible causes of coma. Unless a person's clinical signs rapidly improve — for example, blood glucose levels quickly normalize — a CT scan is vital. Conditions that can be seen on a CT scan include masses, diffuse or multiple brain lesions, water on the brain (edema), bleeding (hemorrhage), fluid buildup deep in the brain (hydrocephalus), shifting of brain tissue, and other indirect signs of increased pressure inside the skull (intracranial pressure).

Sometimes, doctors will refer to abnormalities on a CT scan as densities, and they may point to the degree of grayness and whiteness between areas of the brain. (Density is basically determined by how much radiation appears in an area being

WHAT A CT SCAN CAN REVEAL

- Mass caused by a clot or tumor pressing on other parts and shifting the brain
- Brain swelling on both sides
- Brain edema caused by increased water in the white matter of the brain
- Widening of ventricles caused by filling with fluid or blood
- Major brainstem hemorrhage
- Loss of features and structures caused by a lack of blood and oxygen

scanned.) A physician may use the term *hypodense*, which means less gray, or *hyperdense*, which means more white.

Hypodensity often is an indicator of a stroke or edema. Hypodensity on a CT scan may indicate swelling (edema) in the brain or a mass (tumor). Very low density indicates air, which most often is associated with a penetrating injury. Sometimes, a poorly defined hypodense area may suggest an infection or a collection of pus. Subtle hypodensities in the back (posterior) brain regions may indicate swelling and fluid collections, which may be associated with blood pressure abnormalities related to the coma.

Hyperdensity, meanwhile, suggests bleeding or a blood clot. If an artery has an area of hyperdensity, there's a clot in it.

An abnormality often missed on a CT scan that may account for coma is what's called a hyperdense basilar artery sign. This is a severe blockage (clot) in the artery (basilar artery) that supplies oxygen-rich blood to the brainstem and certain parts of the brain. The condition is uncommon, but should be considered in an individual in acute coma with clinical signs pointing to it. Presence of this sign generally will prompt additional diagnostic tests so that the clot can be retrieved.

When CT scans are performed in individuals seen immediately after cardiac or respiratory resuscitation, lack of oxygen (asphyxia), near drowning, poisoning, and intoxication, the results often are normal. A CT scan isn't sensitive enough to show all ongoing abnormal processes, although we may see abnormalities later, if an individual remains deeply comatose.

MRI findings

MRI is increasingly being used in people who are comatose and it may have value in urgent settings. It's far more revealing than a CT in identifying an injury to the brain related to reduced blood pressure or oxygen. MRI is also better for identifying infection, such as encephalitis or meningitis, as well as documenting acute demyelination.

Finally, MRI is particularly important to view a shift in brain tissue and brainstem displacement. A mass is easy to identify on both CT and MRI scans, but only MRI can reveal its effect on surrounding brain tissue. MRI can quantify the extent of the pressure caused by the mass, indicate the directions of brain shift, demonstrate the possible consequences of compression and document damage.

EEG testing

An electroencephalogram (EEG) can pick up brain activity changes even in individuals who are slightly drowsy and not completely unconscious. EEGs are used to grade the severity of brain injury or brain disease (encephalopathy), usually in patients who have a serious bloodstream infection (sepsis) that has damaged other organs (multiorgan failure).

One of the most interesting patterns physicians see on EEG are periodic

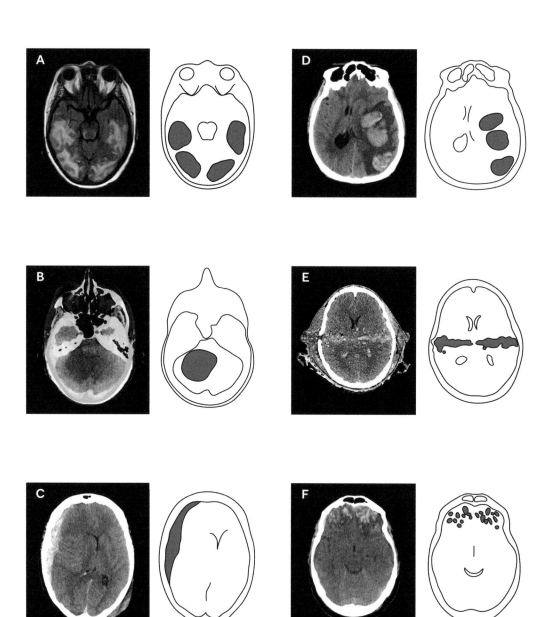

Common findings on CT scans include the following: **A.** Brain swelling in a patient with a high blood pressure surge. **B.** Stroke in the cerebellum that caused major tightness in that compartment. **C.** Blood in the subdural space that caused a brain shift. **D.** Bleeding following a stroke that produced a mass effect. **E.** A gunshot wound through the brain that left a trace of blood and bone fragments. **F.** Bruising in the front of the brain.

lateralized epileptiform discharges and generalized periodic epileptiform discharges. Sharp waves, spikes, slow waves, or a combination are visible. These EEG patterns may present in individuals who have a new brain lesion, and they're common in individuals with viral infections of the brain. When they appear in a constant rhythm, they could be seizures.

The most worrisome EEG pattern is burst-suppression, which usually occurs in patients under deep anesthesia. When it's seen in individuals who aren't sedated, it means that brain function is severely depressed. This happens most often in individuals after experiencing cardiac arrest that severely damaged cortex layers in the brain.

Often, several EEG patterns are seen. Then, the goal is to identify the worst or best ones and the patterns that indicate that an individual's seizures need to be treated immediately. Continuously monitoring comatose patients with EEG for several days may increase early recognition of seizures.

AND FINALLY

It's important to determine the cause of brain injury and review important data from laboratory testing in all people experiencing coma. The findings may be revealing and affect treatment.

In some cases, such as in individuals who are unconscious for a long time before someone finds them and gets them to the

WHAT AN EEG CAN REVEAL

- Slowing of pattern (very common)
- Burst of activity then silence (during anesthesia or after a major injury to cortex)
- Flat pattern (in brain death)
- Spikes and waves (seizures)
- Abnormal wave contours (nonspecific; may be caused by many diseases)

hospital, it may take a while to draw a definitive conclusion. In rare cases, the cause of a coma may remain unknown, but often it's eventually found.

It's not uncommon for individuals experiencing coma to have more than one medical condition. As you'll learn in subsequent chapters of this book, once a major cause is found, it immediately leads to treatment. How quickly treatment occurs and the extent of treatment may determine an individual's future prognosis.

3

How is coma treated?

A CONVERSATION

Physician: This is a CT scan of your father's brain that shows a large blood clot. The clot is pushing on parts of the brain, which may become damaged if we don't do something right away.

Family: Is the bleeding why he's in a coma?

Physician: Yes. We need to ask a neurosurgeon to get the clot out to create more space, and they may remove a piece of your father's skull to make room in case his brain swells more later. We may also give him drugs to reduce the brain swelling.

Family: After that, will he get better?

Physician: We think his brain function will improve, but the recovery may be a long road with a lot of bumps along the way. Because he'll be on long-term bed rest, he may develop complications. Some of them can be life-threatening. We'll watch for any changes in his condition and continue to treat him as things evolve.

Coma is undeniably a major medical emergency. Comatose patients need care that must be rendered quickly. Although not always the case, in many situations the faster the intervention, often the better the outcome. Faced with an individual who is comatose, physicians often don't have the luxury of sitting back and thinking through every decision. They need to know what to do and act on it, or make an immediate referral to someone (preferably a neurointensivist or neurohospitalist) experienced in handling complex, highly acute situations.

Split-second decisions can still be very good decisions, particularly if they're made by experienced physicians. Close relatives and family members of an individual in a coma shouldn't be left in the dark about these decisions. They should be engaged right from the start because patients who are delirious or unconscious clearly don't have the capacity to understand their situations. Their families are truly essential early on to give medical professionals direction about how much care to provide. This can range from using all available measures, to stopping short of performing major surgery, to doing nothing when there's no chance of recovery. As I will repeat over and over in this book, the choice is dependent upon the stated wishes of the individual who's comatose — as expressed in a legal document (health care directive) or during prior conversations with family.

The old approach of "Do what you need to do, doctor" has been replaced with a new approach: "We're planning to [fill in the details and potential consequences of the intervention and treatment], and we're asking for your consent." Only if they can't reach the family does the health care team caring for a comatose patient make decisions regarding treatment. This is viewed as a reasonable emergency exception to informed consent in a critically ill person on the verge of death or at risk of crippling permanent afflic- tion if something isn't done immediately.

No one should be denied urgent medical care because they're too incapacitated to consent or family isn't present. It follows naturally that the team caring for such a patient is expected to act in a manner that will provide the maximum possible benefit and the best outcome.

As I noted in Chapter 2, there are several mechanisms of acute brain injury that can lead to a deep coma. Common causes include a drug overdose, brain trauma and interrupted blood flow, as well as swelling, infection, ongoing seizures and severe blood abnormalities. Some of these conditions can be quite destructive, and little can be done to treat them. In addition, each of these abnormalities can lead to brain swelling, adding more trauma to an already injured organ, particularly the brainstem. Depending on the nature of the injury, an individual's outcome may deviate markedly from what we might expect, and they can be further disabled if another injury occurs.

Once medical staff intervene, acutely comatose patients rarely awaken magically, and these individuals remain in a state of vulnerability. After brain surgery, some leave the operating room only to make a U-turn to undergo another surgery. And patients who seem stable may not be stable, so constant vigilance is required to identify signs of change or deterioration.

An estimated 1 in 3 patients with trauma to the brain will get worse after initial treatment. That's a very high proportion. Remember, these individuals are critically ill, so there's a real and immediate risk that their clinical condition will decline. This can also occur during transfers between medical facilities.

Sending a comatose patient to a medical center without a neurosurgeon on call or an available neurointensivist not only may delay appropriate treatment but may result in a worse outcome if the person needs to be moved again. In some cases, transporting a patient by helicopter rather than by ground can make a major difference, reducing time to get to an operating room by hours. Another benefit of helicopter transport is more rapid application of medical procedures and the availability of a large number of emergency drugs.

Early efforts to stabilize someone who's comatose may include intubation to protect the airway and aid breathing, and steps to treat low or high blood pressure, blood loss, and abnormal blood values. This critical juncture often determines whether a person's condition will improve or decline.

In this chapter, I will explain the options for treating coma, how and why decisions about treatment are made, and what the road ahead may look like. I will also discuss the so-called "golden hour" of treatment. That's the time when prompt medical and surgical actions are most likely to prevent a bad outcome. We'll also discuss complications. While there are standards for treating complications, in very young or very old individuals, we may deviate from them at times. Often, we need to weigh the specifics of the case to decide on the best approach.

Treating an individual in a coma can be daunting. Of course, the health care staff wants a good outcome for every patient. One could convincingly argue that an early, very aggressive approach — trying every means to treat the injury — is warranted and that we should only hold back when there's no success despite every effort.

Some brain injuries, however, can't be treated, no matter what we try. There's simply no way some individuals will improve, often leaving them with a devastating disability. A few of them may never awaken from their coma.

But for many other patients, there are very good options, and it's our job to help them recover.

EARLY TREATMENT

The classic resuscitation ABCs (*Airway, Breathing, Circulation*) or extended ABCDEs (*Airway* with cervical spine protection, *Breathing, Circulation, Disability* and *Exposure* and *Environment*) apply to anyone seen in an emergency setting for the first time. However, these vital signs have special importance in patients with an acute brain injury leading to coma, beyond what they mean in other individuals who are ill.

In many comatose patients, neurologic injury makes it impossible for them to keep their airways open. As a result, they may have very superficial breathing and abnormal breathing rhythms. For that reason alone (and less commonly because of worsening lung function), individuals in a coma are placed on a ventilator. Blood circulation, meanwhile, often remains normal in comatose individuals with acute neurologic injury, unless they've lost all brain function and their blood pressure is unstable. Low blood pressure in acute brain injury is a different story; the cause may be bleeding from another source.

Once we know what we're dealing with, effective treatment often is available. When caring for a comatose individual, physicians often ask themselves and the medical team the following questions.

- *Is the coma caused by a blocked large artery to the brainstem, and can we unblock it?* Clots in the basilar artery are rare, but often they can be retrieved with a very small catheter (the size of a sharp pencil point) or sucked out. The improvement that follows is dramatic. A blocked brainstem artery always should be considered because the window for successful treatment closes quickly.
- *Does the bleeding or tumor have a mass effect?* Bleeding in the brain or a rapidly expanding tumor can compromise other regions, and the pressure created must be rapidly relieved. To do that, we use medication that reduces swelling, or we open the patient's skull and remove the mass. Some of these surgeries are comparatively simple and experienced neurosurgeons don't hesitate to perform them. They include removing a clot located under or on top of the dura — a three-layer membrane attached to the inner surface of the skull — that's pressing on the brain.
- *Does the patient's CT scan show a very large ventricle compartment?* If that's the case, circulation of cerebrospinal fluid has been blocked and a drain must be placed emergently to prevent the individual from rapidly getting worse.
- *Does the patient have a brain infection?* If a brain infection is likely, we immediately treat an individual with antibiotics and antiviral medication without waiting for test results. (If test results are normal, we stop the medications.)
- *Did the patient take a drug overdose or is there a chemical imbalance?* In the case of overdose, if there's an antidote, we give it to the patient. This works the best when the drug is an opioid (heroin) or a benzodiazepine ("benzos"). If a patient's coma was caused by a chemical imbalance, we correct it. Very low blood sugar (glucose) is common, and it's the first test that EMTs administer when they encounter a comatose individual. They usually give glucose to a patient who's been taking insulin, without waiting for results of blood tests. If coma is caused by organ failure other than the brain, the organ's function may need to be taken over by a machine, such as dialysis, in the case of kidney failure.
- *Is the patient having seizures?* If a comatose individual is seizing, a single infusion of a high-dose anti-epileptic medication may be effective and should be given immediately, without hesitation. This is particularly true if one seizure follows another.
- *Is the patient hypothermic?* In rare circumstances, coma occurs because of a steep drop in core body temperature. When this happens, an individual may

look stiff and blue and appear dead, but warming them often does wonders. (The saying goes, "You're not dead until you're warm and dead.")

The scenarios I've just described aren't rare. Some are seen every week among patients treated in emergency departments and intensive care units (ICUs). The conditions we see most often are generally the easiest to manage. It's more difficult to sort out treatment for a comatose patient when the cause is odd or something we encounter only occasionally.

In some cases, however, there's a painful realization that treatment and recovery will be prolonged, and the person's true outcome may not be known for months or even years.

MANAGING COMPLICATIONS

Our next priority is treating complications, both in the brain and the rest of the body.

For the family of a patient in a coma, it can be very frustrating to hear a physician say, "Everything was going in the right direction, but your loved one has had a serious setback."

Among older patients, the new injury may restart previous health problems. Systemic triggers, such as marked hypoxemia, high blood carbon dioxide or hypotension, can be potentially damaging, so aggressive steps should be taken to manage them. Hypotension can also occur in individuals who develop an infection that evolves into sepsis.

Among individuals with a traumatic brain injury, other trauma may cause instability. In some cases, use of anesthetic drugs can trigger a significant drop in blood pressure (hypotension). Sedation carries the risk of low oxygen or high carbon dioxide due to upper airway obstruction. Simple procedures to open the windpipe (trachea) such as a tracheostomy can cause a sudden change in blood pressure

URGENT COMA INTERVENTIONS THAT MAY PRODUCE RAPID RESULTS

- Removal of a clot in the basilar artery
- Surgical removal of a blood clot pressing on the brain
- Drainage of enlarged ventricles
- Treatment of acute brain infection with antibiotics or antiviral drugs
- Administration of an antidote to drug intoxication
- Administration of anti-seizure medications
- Dialysis for kidney shutdown
- Supplementation for thyroid failure
- Warming measures for hypothermia

or oxygenation that may tip a patient already in a delicate balance over the edge.

It's also not uncommon for comatose patients to get worse, even after the inciting trigger has been treated. Complications that occur later on after recovery, such as dealing with a disability, are discussed in Chapter 5.

Neurologic complications: The brain under pressure

Treatment to relieve increased brain (intracranial) pressure is quite common among patients with a brain injury. As I explain how pressure can build inside the brain, keep the following image in mind.

Think of the skull as a closed box with the brain inside. A healthy brain is a floppy mass beneath the skull. Two things are necessary to maintain its shape: 1) pulsating blood and cerebrospinal fluid flowing through it; and 2) the presence of several compartments. The left side of the brain is separated from the right by a hard structure that doesn't stretch or expand easily and mostly stays in place.

Arteries provide blood to the brain, and veins take blood away from the brain. Cerebrospinal fluid surrounds the brain and enters natural cavities inside the brain. Cerebrospinal fluid not only is a shock absorber, it also provides nourishment and removes waste. All these parts help to regulate pressure underneath the skull. Inside the brain, the pressure is low — usually in the single digits, measured in millimeters of mercury.

As I mentioned in Chapter 1, increased pressure causes the brain to shift, sometimes from one compartment to the other (herniation). The result is more brain in one compartment, where it doesn't belong, than in the other, causing increased pressure. About 10% of your brain is made up of blood, cerebrospinal fluid makes up another 10% and the brain itself accounts for 80% of the space beneath the skull.

The brain consists mostly of water, and an important law of physics is that water is nearly incompressible. So new volume due to swelling or a clot can't be easily accommodated for. Even an increase in brain volume of less than 10% is serious in a young person. Unfortunately, nature has very few ways to compensate for that.

Too much pressure pushes blood from inside the brain out into the veins. Fluids may be pushed out of the brain into the spine. Pressure rises exponentially, which means that a small increase in volume will cause a much larger increase in pressure, and the cycle continues until the pressure is very high.

Among older adults (age causes the brain to shrink) or in patients with a prior injury or stroke that's resulted in loss of brain substance, the patient can tolerate increased volume, and the steep curve flattens out, but not by much. Eventually, the pressure rises unrelentingly.

As you can imagine, high pressure beneath the skull compresses all the structures inside it until they stop functioning. That's one reason why we lose consciousness. Unfortunately, when the pressure is sustained, the brain doesn't snap back. Lack of blood flow from increased pressure leads to death in parts of the brain that don't receive enough blood. This occurs in addition to an injury the patient already may have experienced.

A major principle in acute neurology is that increased pressure will further damage the brain, sometimes permanently, and certainly if it involves the brainstem, which is where all the vital functions reside. Therefore, we must find a way to reduce the pressure.

Following are the most important interventions to reduce intracranial pressure. Other routine measures also may be taken, such as temperature control, blood pressure control, monitoring of oxygen and carbon dioxide levels, and positioning the head of the bed at a 30-degree angle.

Drains

A simple way to relieve pressure is to insert a catheter into the brain's fluid compartments and remove fluid. However, if the swelling is significant, these compartments are already compressed and narrowed, and it's difficult to remove fluid from a tight brain.

Sometimes, the ventricles enlarge because blood prevents fluids from being absorbed. This also causes increased pressure, but in this situation, the pressure can be relieved by draining the fluid. The body produces about 30 cubic centimeters of cerebrovascular fluid every hour, and

draining approximately the same amount allows us to keep pressure in check. We see this used in patients with ruptured cerebral aneurysms.

Medication

Another option is to shrink the brain with medication. Over many years, we've found that administering highly concentrated sugar or salt causes water in the brain to move into circulation by way of a simple osmosis mechanism (see the illustration on page 60).

Hyperconcentrated saline or sugar alcohols are quite effective for this purpose, acting as a sponge and sucking up enormous amounts of brain fluid very rapidly. After a single dose of mannitol (the standard sugar alcohol), a patient may wake up or exhibit signs — such as the pupil of an eye reacting to light — indicating improvement in brain compression.

Many physicians will give mannitol to patients when they anticipate brain swelling and even before a CT scan is ordered. In fact, hyperconcentrated saline and sugar alcohols are among our most important tools to quickly reduce increased brain pressure.

Surgery

One more option is to "open the box" with surgery. About half the bone that makes up the skull is removed to quickly relieve the pressure. This is standard procedure in patients with a blood clot on top of or inside the brain that needs to be removed surgically.

This procedure, called hemicraniectomy, is performed in an operating room under anesthesia. During the procedure, half of the skull is removed and stored in a freezer. Obviously, this is a major surgery with risks of infection and wound leakage. Additional surgery is required, months later after the patient has improved, to replace the missing bone, and sometimes during that procedure, mesh material is added.

Monitors

Pressure inside the brain can be measured with a pressure monitor placed directly into brain tissue. Many ICUs have these devices. We regularly check the pressure level and try to keep it as low as possible.

Pressure monitors may be used in patients who've already lapsed into a deep coma due to increased intracranial pressure. To date, monitors are the only way to measure pressure inside the brain. The search for a noninvasive bedside monitor has

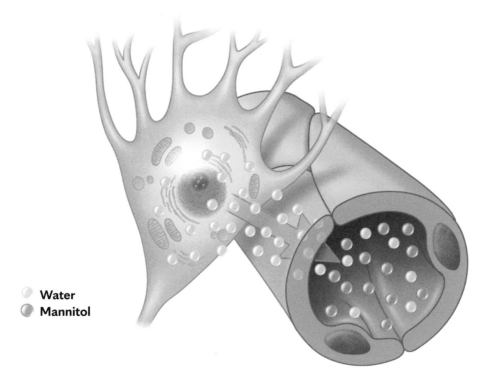

- Water
- Mannitol

In this illustration of a brain cell and artery, highly concentrated sugars (mannitol) shrink brain tissues by soaking up brain water entering the artery by way of osmosis.

been compared with a search for the Holy Grail.

Medications, drainage of fluid and surgery all can be helpful for treating brain swelling. Other measures such as treating fever, lowering blood pressure and controlling glucose also can help, but there's always the risk the condition will become overwhelming, because the brain has so little room to compensate for the swelling. Once the brain is overwhelmed, we rapidly run out of options.

As a last resort, surgeons sometimes remove some brain tissue to create more space, but in general, this should be avoided.

Neurologic complications: Seizures

A fair number of individuals in a coma have seizures. Bleeding deep in the brain seldom causes seizures. Frequently, they're the result of irritation to neurons located on the surface of the brain. Seizures can occur soon after an individual arrives at the hospital, but we usually see them 24 hours after the event that led to the coma or after surgery. A patient who fails to awaken after emergency surgery might be actively seizing. Fortunately, this happens much less often than we're led to believe or can demonstrate.

Seizures can cause a patient's eyes to turn to one side and an eyelid, the chin or an arm to twitch rhythmically. These movements are fleeting and may disappear by the time a nurse or physician walks into the room. Some individuals appear to have brief moments of eye contact and responsiveness and then look spaced out or blank. A prolonged (12- to 24-hour) EEG can capture passing seizures. If we find seizures, we treat them, but unfortunately, that doesn't always lead to improvement. Seizures may indicate additional, perhaps uncurable, brain injury, and treatment may not help.

Seizures can occur regardless of what caused the coma. They're more common, however, in individuals who've overdosed. A classic seizure is often obvious. After first stiffening, the person's muscles jerk rhythmically. The eyes may roll sideways or upward. If the person isn't on a ventilator breathing may become very irregular, and the individual may gasp and make loud noises.

Protecting an individual from harm during seizures (such as with padded bedrails and a mouthguard) is essential. Otherwise, the tongue may be significantly damaged, and it may swell and obstruct the airway later. Medications given intravenously can block seizures, but there's a fine line to walk with that treatment.

Good, early responsiveness to medication is what we want. Lack of response may lead to use of additional medications, leaving a patient "under" (sedated) a long time. If recovery occurs, it will likely be prolonged.

Unmanageable (therapy-refractory) seizures remain a major neurologic complication of coma, and they can affect a patient's outcome in a very bad way.

TREATING PROLONGED COMA

Many individuals who are comatose awaken. If that doesn't occur or a patient doesn't improve as well or as quickly as was expected, additional treatments may be considered. One of the first things we do is try to reduce or eliminate any medications that may be hindering an individual's awareness. We determine which medications are absolutely necessary and which aren't.

For patients in a minimally conscious state, use of antidepressants, amphetamines (such as Ritalin, which improves processing speed, attention and possibly memory) and implantation of electrical leads in the brain (deep brain stimulation) have been studied. But the results of these approaches have been disappointing.

The drug amantadine is the only medical intervention that seems to benefit individuals in a minimally conscious state. In a clinical trial, it was given for four weeks to individuals who had been injured one to four months beforehand. The group receiving the medication showed faster recovery on disability scales.

However, we don't know whether amantadine has longer-term benefits. The study also hasn't been replicated by other investigators to prove its benefit. This has relevance for patients in a prolonged coma after traumatic brain injury, in whom the course of improvement may be prolonged, transiently stall and then improve again. Recovery from coma is often unpredictable, in particular in young adults and children.

A particular concern for families is that when coma starts to lift, their loved ones may begin to experience unpleasant symptoms. However, we don't think that patients experience any emotional consequences of pain, even if they show physiological signs — loud moaning or crying, tensing up, flushing and repeated grimacing — that suggest distress. Pain is a primitive response, and some patients in a minimally conscious state apparently respond to pain and may be able to perceive it. In this situation, physicians may prescribe pain relief medications, if only to reassure nursing staff, families and perhaps even themselves.

The overriding theme is the scarcity of options for individuals in a prolonged coma. Medications and stimulating methods just don't work. For many patients and families, the best approach is simply time, which physicians refer to as watchful waiting, along with continued medical support and surveillance for complications. We know the condition of someone in a coma can change, and quite a few people in a minimally conscious state become more responsive and start to speak single words. That endpoint may still be a very significant disability that can be challenging for caregivers. Patients themselves may be more frustrated than distressed by the awareness that they have a major neurologic handicap.

Medical complications

Once we've optimized a patient's brain function ("brain-resuscitated" the patient), we enter a wait-and-see mode and intervene when needed. During this time, the concerns are complications associated with immobilization and critical care support.

Risks associated with lying in bed are more severe than those of taking a long flight or long road trip. Immobilization is very dangerous, and with each passing day, something can happen. Also, being on a ventilator, though necessary to ensure adequate oxygen, isn't good for the lungs. Unnatural stretching and pressure may cause lung injury and formation of mucous plugs. Patients on ventilators also require drugs that cause irregular fast or slow heart rhythms on an already stressed heart. In my experience, some families don't appreciate these tremendous risks and assume that good nursing care will pull their loved one through, but complications are inevitable.

There are two types of complications: anticipated and unanticipated. Anticipated complications are related to long-term bed rest and immobilization. Minimal limb movement, including paralysis, is a major risk. Unanticipated complications are rare but more common among patients with preexisting medical conditions. Preexisting conditions can flare when the body is under enormous stress. Unanticipated complications could be a heart attack, development of diabetes, bleeding in the stomach or an embolism in a lung. A prolonged coma makes a person extremely vulnerable to these and other setbacks.

Unanticipated complications are often overlooked in initial discussions with

families about their loved ones' possible outcomes. Unanticipated complications are generally best tolerated (and survived) by young, healthy individuals and are a cause for great concern among those who are older and fragile. Anything can happen. For example, we may find an advanced cancer in a patient who has a stroke resulting in a coma.

Optimal supportive care includes:
- *Providing nutrition.* Tubes that carry food and fluids to the stomach through the nose (nasogastric tubes) are used to ensure comatose patients receive adequate nutrition. A standard enteral formula or a calorically dense formula is sufficient. When coma is prolonged, an individual may receive nutrition through a tube that's surgically placed in the stomach (gastrostomy). This is a safer option.
- *Tending to the eyes, mouth and skin.* Vaseline or lip balm protects the lips from dryness and cracking.
- *Frequent mouth sponging. Candida albicans* is a fungus that's part of the normal flora in the gastrointestinal tract, but individuals who are critically ill and comatose can experience an overgrowth, which can be treated.
- *Managing body fluids.* Tissues may swell over time because of the large amounts of fluids a patient receives.
- *Bowel care and monitoring for nonfunctioning bowels.* Bowel care includes keeping the person's skin clean and dry. Among comatose patients, diarrhea can have many causes, but often it's related to certain nutritional formulas and can be resolved by changing the fiber content. Antibiotics

or bacterial infections such as *Escherichia coli* and *Clostridium difficile* also can cause diarrhea. Failure to pass stool or passing marble-like stools should be treated with a rectal enema. Marked abdominal swelling (distention) is an early sign of nonfunctioning bowels.

- *Urinary care.* Indwelling catheters are required in comatose patients. It's important to monitor the patient for urinary tract infections, which are common in individuals needing urinary catheters for a long period of time. The use of diapers, pads or condom catheters may promote colonization of bacteria and skin breakdown.
- *Prevention of blood clots in the legs.* The risk of deep vein thrombosis (DVT) is much higher in someone with a traumatic head injury who's undergone major surgery than in an individual whose coma is associated with drug intoxication, for example. DVT is also more common in patients with leg weakness, which increases blood pooling due to limited muscle contractions to drive circulation. We often inject heparin to prevent this.
- *Preventing and treating bedsores.* Another concern is the development of bedsores (decubitus ulcers). Bedsores are even more likely in patients transferred to a long-term care facility. Nursing staff take steps to reduce their occurrence by repositioning the patient's body, but bedsores are inevitable among patients in a prolonged coma. There's very little evidence that certain support surfaces can reduce their development; however, air-fluid beds may be used to try to reduce their numbers or severity.

- *Reducing the risk of new infections.* Lung infections can develop in patients after even short periods on a mechanical ventilator, and some can become serious and enter the bloodstream, causing sepsis. The most common health care-related infections in comatose individuals are those that occur in the lungs and the urinary tract, and those associated with catheters placed in large veins.

Antibiotic-resistant infections

Resistance of bacteria to antibiotics has increased tremendously and complicated treatment. Over the last decade, several classes of antibiotics have become ineffective in treating new infections. Comatose individuals are at high risk of hospital-acquired pneumonia — an estimated 40% to 70% incidence with a traumatic brain injury.

Individuals in a prolonged coma who've been exposed to multiple antibiotics and are older than age 60 are at greatest risk of severe infection from antibiotic-resistant pathogens. That is why medical staff follow strict guidelines for infection control, including putting on a gown before gloving, changing gloves to prevent cross-contamination of different body sites, and sanitizing their hands after they remove their gloves and gown.

Storming

A fever is most often associated with an infection, but fever may also be an indicator of a condition referred to as storming.

The medical term for this condition is paroxysmal sympathetic hyperactivity syndrome. Storming frequently goes unrecognized and untreated. Storming spells are most common in young patients with a traumatic brain injury but can occur after any major brain injury.

In addition to fever, symptoms include a rapid heart rate, increased breathing, profound sweating and stiffening up. Patients who are storming may also develop severe jaw clenching and teeth grinding. Effective treatments for the condition include the use of morphine and high doses of the anticonvulsant medication gabapentin.

Tracheostomy

Most individuals who remain comatose are intubated and placed on mechanical ventilation. After two weeks, if the patient can't be easily weaned from intubation, a tracheostomy may be considered. This procedure facilitates breathing by creating an opening in the neck with windpipe access. The benefit of a tracheostomy is better airway clearance.

Pulmonary embolism

An individual in a coma who develops rapid breathing (tachypnea) or a rapid heartbeat (tachycardia) may have a blood clot in a lung (pulmonary embolism). A scan of the chest arteries may help to find the embolism. High-intensity blood thinners are generally used to treat the condition. Treatment may also include

placing of a filter into a large vein to prevent clots in the individual's legs from migrating to the lungs.

PHYSICAL THERAPY TO PREVENT CONTRACTURE

It's important to begin physical therapy early and to focus attention on the positioning of the limbs. Increased muscle tension is expected with a severe brain injury, and the result is quick stiffening of the limbs. This can lead to shortening of the muscles and fixed positions that can't be overcome with movement or stretching. The end result is muscle contracture — tightening and shortening of the muscles, leading to deformity.

Studies have shown comatose patients who receive fewer than four sessions per week of physical therapy are more likely to experience muscle contracture than those who receive at least four sessions.

Several physical therapy techniques are used to counteract contracture, such as specific positioning of limbs, feet and fingers (in bed and later in a medical chair); splinting and even casting, and passive range-of-movement exercises to avoid rapid deterioration of normal movement.

If contracture isn't treated and a coma-tose patient awakens and becomes more mobile, stiff joints may complicate the patient's rehabilitation and make it impossible to get out of a wheelchair. That's why positioning of the joints and range of movement should be very much on a physician's radar screen from day one.

Initial care involves physiotherapy, and it should start as soon as treatment won't be functionally disruptive. Studies have shown that the impact of passive range of motion — the patient is passive, and the physical therapist moves the limbs and stretches the muscles — has no harmful effect on heart rate, respiratory rate, blood pressure or pressure inside the brain. This is true in individuals who are breathing spontaneously as well as those on mechanical ventilation, regardless of the cause of a coma.

Early use of stretching exercises can help individuals who've been in a coma only a short time to maintain range of motion. Gentle, passive range of motion and stretching are the techniques most often used. Therapies such as electrical stimulation, ultrasound and botulinum toxin injections, alone or in combination, have been shown to provide only limited, and short-term, effects. There's evidence, however, that 30 minutes of a soft-splint application reduces spasticity and improves hand-opening in some individuals. The individuals tolerate soft splinting well, and it's a technique that doesn't require supervision.

Virtually all individuals in a vegetative state eventually develop lower-limb contractures. Motions in the upper limbs may prevent contracture, but the spastic state of legs in a vegetative state for months is so profound that it invariably leads to contractures. Unfortunately, no physical therapy program has been able to prevent major contractures in patients in a prolonged coma. They eventually develop bent (flexion) contractures in their elbows, wrists and fingers, in which the joint cannot be straightened. The legs become rigid, and the feet take on a position similar to that of a classic ballet stance.

AND FINALLY

Caring for an individual who's comatose is complex and requires the skills of a multidisciplinary team that includes neuroscience nursing staff, pharmacists who specialize in intensive care drugs, respiratory therapists who specialize in ventilator management, social workers, chaplains and so on. Other physicians, such as a neurosurgeon, nephrologist and infectious disease specialist, also may be involved.

In recent years, treatment options in intensive care have changed quite dramatically, and we've also realized the importance of early intervention in giving patients a chance for survival and successful rehabilitation.

Daily care involves continuous monitoring of every organ system (see the table on the opposite page). During morning rounds, not only do we discuss an individual's neurologic condition ("Has there been any change?"), but we also go over in detail the state of every organ system.

The body is complex, and the sum is more than its parts. In medicine, however, we try to isolate smaller systems, look at them first, and then apply what we've learned on a broader level, considering how everything is connected and how treatment for one condition can affect another.

Treatment involves both short- and long-term care. Immediately treating the primary cause of a coma is essential, but afterward an individual may enter a difficult period and experience major complications. Efforts to prevent and treat complications are equally essential. It's no exaggeration to say we must tread carefully with all potential complications associated with acute brain injury.

OTHER CONCERNS IN COMATOSE PATIENTS

Organ system	Concern or treatment
Lungs	• Mechanical ventilation • Tracheostomy care • Infection surveillance
Heart	• Irregular heart rate • EKG changes • Blood pressure regulation
Gastrointestinal	• Preventive measures to protect stomach • Nutrition and choice of formula • Glucose/insulin drips • Motility of bowels (assistance)
Bladder	• Catheter care • Monitoring for infection
Eyes/mouth/skin	• Eye protection • Prevention and treatment of bed sores • Mouthwashes
Medication	• Need for and choice of antibiotics • Blood thinners to prevent blood clots in legs • Avoidance of major drug-drug interactions • Assessment of need for ongoing sedation and analgesia

When can we expect awakening and recovery?

A CONVERSATION

Physician: We've noticed improvement in your daughter, and I'm sure you have, too. When you said she was opening her eyes briefly and looking at you, I wasn't so sure. But now it's clear that she's coming around and more awake and likely aware.

Family: How do we know she'll be fine? What should we look for when we visit her?

Physician: The first and most important signs to watch for are her looking around; in particular, keeping a focus on people in the room.

Family: How much longer will it be before she recognizes us?

Physician: It will be very gradual, and there will be days when nothing much happens and other days when she'll make good strides. Of course, each patient's trajectory of improvement is different.

When recovery does happen, it's generally in stages. First, the person awakens and then becomes aware and begins to communicate. Later, the individual becomes more energetic, dynamic and focused, and acquires motivation to reach new physical and mental objectives and goals.

None of these stages is predictable, let alone clearly outlined, and they're mostly unrelated to the cause of a coma. During early recovery of a comatose individual, medical staff often is careful to avoid labeling the severity of the patient's condition so as not to affect the level of care the person receives. Sometimes, computerized tomography (CT) scans may not look good, but the patient is better than the scans suggest, and we need to rely on neurologic examinations to determine progress or lack thereof.

THE UNKNOWNS OF RECOVERY

A few things regarding coma and recovery we know. We know that a single shot of a so-called antidote can reverse many comas related to an intentional or unintentional drug overdose. As we've seen during the opioid epidemic, naloxone induces an almost miraculous awakening in individuals who've overdosed on opioids. The same thing may occur when flumazenil is given to someone who's taken too many benzodiazepine pills, such as valium or other anti-anxiety medications, but this effect is less dramatic.

Unfortunately, not every individual who receives one of these antidotes recovers. A prolonged period of very low oxygen levels and reduced blood pressure can leave its mark.

Over the years, several important observations have been made about patients who emerge from their comas. Severe injury to the brain doesn't disappear overnight; it may be weeks before an individual's injured brain improves to the point the person seems to "come to the surface." Another important insight is that family members often see more changes in a

loved one and earlier on than do nursing staff and physicians. In part, this is due to family members' constant attentiveness at the bedside, but it's also because they know the loved one best and, thus, are more likely to notice an attempt to make contact. We take that very seriously and follow up when it occurs.

Other changes in comatose individuals may not necessarily have much meaning. One is opening the eyes. This is only meaningful if there's so-called fixation; that is, the patient's eyes briefly but repeatedly look at something or someone in the room, such as a family member or a nurse who's approaching. It also may occur when the patient is asked to do a specific task (for example, "look to the left," "look upward"). Unfortunately, eye-opening triggered by stimulation — in response to an auditory startle, such as a loud noise made above the individual's head — may not mean much and even occurs in individuals who remain in a coma for prolonged periods.

Open eyes are often greeted by family as an awakening or a major improvement, but as I mentioned in Chapter 1, it's difficult to come to grips with a blank stare that's void of any eye contact. In this situation, most families agree that their loved ones are "not there," aren't able to think independently, and aren't participating in social interaction.

In this chapter, I review the trajectories of improvement in comatose patients, but please don't assume these trajectories are predictable or fixed. During recovery from an acute brain injury, nothing can be predicted with certainty, and we shouldn't harbor illusions. Nothing is predestined when it comes to neurologic recovery. No reliable tool can estimate the recovery of consciousness after coma. Recovery remains somewhat mysterious biologically, but we're glad for it when it occurs. Many people recover after being in a coma, even if they've been comatose for some time. Recovery isn't a cure, but it surely counts for something.

For the most part, comatose patients who awaken quickly generally do well. Outcomes are often worse among individuals who remain comatose for longer periods. Outcomes may include limited resilience, cognitive deficits and lack of physical reserves. Given the mixed picture and many variables, physicians often are forced to consider what defines quality of life and whether to recommend aggressive treatment.

For sure, recovery in patients who are comatose often is K shaped. At a certain point the paths of the individuals diverge, like the arms of the letter K, with some on a relentlessly downward trajectory and others going up and improving daily.

The path a patient may take often is unpredictable, and time is needed to map out the true trajectory. In individuals with

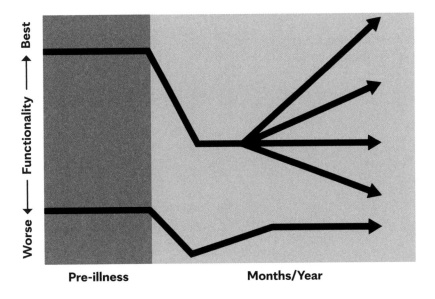

This graph shows several possible trajectories among comatose patients who had high functionality before their injuries and experienced rapid declines after losing consciousness. As you can see, some may regain all the functionality they once had. Others will improve, but not back to their baselines. And for some their functioning may become much worse. Patients who had poor functionality before their illness may improve but typically never beyond their baseline levels.

histories of poor health, recovery may occur, but these individuals may have much less functionality over the long term.

This book's starting point is that coma resulting from a brain injury lays bare a major (and sometimes tragic) medical concern, and we may have to wait to know the outcome. However, over time, comatose patients often provide indications that they are improving or when things are likely to turn around, as shown in the shaded boxes below.

EARLY SIGNS OF IMPROVEMENT

One of the first indications of improvement we see is increased movement. For example, a patient who exhibited only reflex movements, such as stiffening up or bending at the elbow, now knows where on the body he or she is being touched and may move an arm up to the area that's being pinched. This action shows a sense of purpose, indicating a relatively high degree of active brain function.

Once that target is achieved, further improvement may happen next. After purposeful localization of a pinch, fine finger movements may occur, and an individual may be able to squeeze a hand and, eventually, give a sign. Once a patient responds to a simple task, such as "Show me two fingers," "Give me a peace sign," or "Give me a thumbs-up (or thumbs-down) sign," we're on a good trajectory and can expect full awakening and participation. Often, this coincides with an individual being able to look at a person repeatedly (fixating) or follow an object up and down with the eyes (tracking).

At this stage, the individual often can't make sounds or speak intelligibly.

ENCOURAGING OUTCOMES AND INDICATORS

- Quick recognition and elimination of the bacteria or virus
- Ability to remove a clot
- Ability to relieve brain swelling
- Rapid improvement within days of medical treatment or surgery
- No prolonged seizures
- No neurologic findings other than impaired consciousness
- No major complications or setbacks
- Good prior health

STAGES IN COMA RECOVERY

- Visual fixation and tracking
- Reacting to a task
- Holding an object
- Recovered ability to speak
- Recovered ability to communicate
- Increased alertness
- Beginning of consistency and reproducibility of actions

Noticeable progress in that area is often hampered by a tracheostomy, which makes speech impossible without a special tube (cannula). Lip movements are often difficult to interpret; they may or may not indicate that an individual is trying to say something. A patient emerging from a coma sometimes displays verbalization. The person might speak a single word or answer yes and no.

Often, the next step is for the individual to hold an object, such as a ball. Eventually, the individual will be able to imitate the proper use of objects, such as using a comb for grooming and using a tooth-brush for cleaning teeth. At this point, the person becomes very aware of his or her surroundings and is on a trajectory of further improvement. The person may proceed from having the ability to move from the bed to a chair, to standing, and eventually, walking with assistance.

An often-difficult road

During recovery, we as physicians must manage expectations very carefully. Unfortunately, awakening and becoming more aware often are associated with loss of some intellectual function, skills, strength and dexterity.

In addition, individuals may have vision difficulties, such as seeing only part of the visual field or seeing double. Some vision issues can be corrected with surgery or prism glasses, but these issues tend to be overlooked. Surprisingly, they're not included in scales for rating outcomes of recovered comatose patients.

A severe brain injury increases the potential for depression and apathy, which may be interrupted by episodes of aggressive behavior and panic attacks. A patient's response to other people may be significantly impaired. The patient might forget easily, have a very low tolerance for stressful situations and be unable to multitask. Among older adults who may already have been challenged in the digital world, electronic devices can rapidly become overwhelming. Given all this frustration, patients emerging from coma may be less able to control their behaviors or keep up with the rapidly changing digital world, increasing their risks of social isolation, loneliness and helplessness.

People seldom appreciate how much we rely on our emotions to function in the world. Emotions give us powerful and critical feedback. People who survive severe comas caused by traumatic brain injuries are at risk of addiction. Their moral alarm bell ("Don't do it!") doesn't go off. Many of these individuals need close follow-up and support through the recovery period, which may take years. Many addiction experts now operate on the assumption that addiction isn't a moral or discipline failure, but rather a brain disorder that may carry a genetic predisposition.

It's important to emphasize that the long-term outcome for coma survivors is a moving target. Indeed, a patient who makes it out of the hospital may look much different a year later. The sad fact is, however, that if an individual's functional independence entails being able to take care of only basic needs, the person's quality of life may not be satisfactory (see Chapter 8). These individuals may have major memory problems, such as the inability to complete familiar tasks. They may get lost while walking or driving in a familiar area, exhibit poor judgment and decision-making, have difficulty with conversation, misplace things, and not recognize family members — all of which may persist for several years or never improve.

Following traumatic brain injuries, some individuals experience ongoing seizures. This is more common in those who've undergone brain surgery to remove a clot or part of the skull to accommodate swelling. Surgical scars may be the source of the seizures, and in many cases, several medications are needed to control them. Unfortunately, remembering to take medication every day can be a formidable task for an individual with memory difficulties or with a lower level of functioning. If medication isn't taken on a regular basis, the seizures may reappear.

The good news is outcomes in younger individuals who've been comatose for several weeks after injuries can be quite spectacular (and even truly miraculous). They may spend a year in a rehabilitation center and reemerge similar mentally and physically to how they were before the injury, with only minor adjustments in their daily functioning.

It's extremely encouraging and, often, quite emotional when our patients return to see us and we see how much progress they've made. The patients may not remember much, but we all immediately remember them and continue to be surprised by the resilience of youth. Even in older adults, the potential exists for delayed but better-than-expected outcomes, with some being able to return to work in their regular jobs, with some adjustments.

RECOVERY FROM A DRUG-INDUCED COMA

In a considerable number of comatose patients, their unconscious states are drug-induced. Some also have a brain injury and marked difficulty with ventilation (rapid, uncontrolled rhythms) or respiration (poor gas exchange). In these people, recovery is largely determined by their brain injuries.

If there's no brain injury — the coma is related to another cause such as a drug overdose or diabetes — a patient's recovery, even after days on a ventilator, is likely to be rapid once the drug or metabolic imbalance is corrected. The patient may be disoriented for several days, to the extent of having hallucinations and delirium, but should soon be back to the prior mental baseline.

Individuals on ventilators for a week or more often lose considerable muscle mass and may have very significant muscle injuries. (We still don't know how this fast-acting damage occurs.) They may have difficulty moving their limbs; in fact, the limbs may not move at all. Some medications, such as the high-dose steroids needed to treat lung disease or drugs to control ventilation, can increase muscle weakness. Reversing muscle deterioration requires a comprehensive physical therapy program with weekly goals for improvement. The process can take several months, but many individuals fully recover their muscle strength.

Delayed awakening from a comatose state can occur if an individual's illness has resulted in organ shutdown, and it takes longer for sedative medications to be cleared from the body. Studies show that drugs given by infusion, such as intravenous (IV) medications, stay in the body longer, and their use may delay full awakening by 1 to 2 weeks. Marked obesity, heart failure and other organ dysfunction also can contribute to prolonged clearance of the medications and their active breakdown products. (We've seen the same thing during the SARS-CoV-2 pandemic in the sickest patients. We don't know whether it's a direct effect of the virus on the brain or due to the often prolonged, tremendously high doses of medications needed to make patients in respiratory distress comfortable on ventilation.)

Waiting and watching is the best approach to individuals who don't awaken right away after being taken off ventilation, and families shouldn't immediately assume something bad has happened.

RECOVERY FROM TRAUMATIC BRAIN INJURY

Approximately 10% to 40% of patients with very severe traumatic brain injuries who are comatose fail to improve and die in the hospital; in some cases, a decision is made to "let a patient go." Among those who survive, recovery varies. However, studies within large databases that contain information about similar cases have provided a much better idea of what to expect in patients with traumatic brain injury in the first months and year(s) after coma.

Of course, some of the data were from patients who had better outcomes because they received inpatient rehabilitation. Factors such as an individual's age, the involvement of a rehabilitation physician and the proximity of the hospital to an inpatient rehabilitation facility play a role in whether an individual who's emerged from a coma is referred for inpatient rehabilitation. In fact, that decision may play an even bigger role than a patient's clinical status in determining whether the patient recovers.

Nearly half the individuals with severe traumatic brain injuries who receive inpatient rehabilitation were initially comatose, and 1 in 10 had some reduction in consciousness when admitted to the hospital. Of course, there's so-called referral bias; that is, individuals who are expected to have better outcomes are more likely to be considered for inpatient rehabilitation.

The main message here, however, is that improvement is possible in a person who has awakened from a coma and has a disturbance of consciousness, roughly defined as not following instructions and dozing off when not stimulated. Whether improved consciousness predicts functional recovery is unclear. And many studies suggest it doesn't. Of patients who are comatose and receive critical care, 40% achieve partial or complete functional independence during rehabilitation. Patients who become comatose while hospitalized and are discharged with low functional status experience greater absolute improvement during rehabilitation.

Outcome after traumatic brain injury is clearly determined by whether a person receives aggressive treatment for increased intracranial pressure, which may include neurosurgery, as described in the previous chapter. Audits of ICUs show that there's substantial variation in the methods used to lower intracranial pressure and marked variation of placement of intracranial monitors.

How long an individual has been comatose is an unreliable predictor of awakening because the person may have been sedated to control agitation or to facilitate mechanical ventilation. Using brain scans to predict prognosis also isn't reliable. I can attest that very disturbing CT scans don't always translate well to the bedside. Some patients with negative findings on imaging do better than others.

Individuals who are severely disabled after a head injury may be able to return to work in sheltered workplaces, usually with reduced duties. The ability to rejoin the workforce and hold a job also may be limited by visual difficulties, nonspecific sensations of vertigo, and panic and fear

attacks that resemble stress reactions. In the first year after a traumatic brain injury, reasoning and responses are often delayed and short-term memory is substantially altered. The result may be less functional independence.

Approximately 3 out of every 4 patients admitted to rehabilitation centers for traumatic brain injuries also have episodes of violent agitation. Depression and apathy can occur together and may respond to medications that simulate brain function. Also, post-traumatic stress disorder and major emotional and behavioral changes can occur in individuals with or without objective findings of brain injury. A comprehensive program is required to treat these issues.

RECOVERY FROM A MAJOR STROKE

A stroke may be caused by a clot inside a brain artery or vein that interrupts blood flow to and away from certain areas of the brain. In either case, brain areas deprived of blood quickly die. A stroke also may result from a clot inside the brain that directly damages brain tissue and places surrounding tissue under increased pressure.

Coma isn't commonly seen in a person who's had a stroke unless: 1) a large clot presses on the other side of the brain or on the brainstem; 2) there's an abnormality deep in the brain and in the brain's thalamus that switches consciousness off and on; or 3) there's a large clot in the brainstem or in the basilar artery that has damaged the cells that spur conscious awareness. I've also seen patients with a previous large stroke in one brain hemisphere who've then become comatose after having another stroke in the opposite hemisphere.

Coma results when both hemispheres of the brain are involved. If function in one hemisphere is restored, the individual awakens, but neurologic problems are present. Other parts of the brain may be able to take over the functions of damaged parts, or at least mitigate some of the injury. We see this in patients with weakness and speech problems. In contrast, some problems, such as double vision, may last for a while or never fully resolve.

A clot in a main brain artery, such as the middle cerebral artery, can lead to a large stroke, with a higher likelihood of swelling. When the swelling is significant, the outcome often is poor, particularly if decompressive hemicraniectomy isn't performed or if it's done in an individual older than age 60. Timing of the procedure — too early or too late — also influences outcome. Not surprisingly, evidence suggests that decompressive surgery done before the patient develops major signs of deterioration is more beneficial than if performed afterward.

Outcomes for patients with smaller hemispheric strokes also depend on the level of neurointensive care that they receive. Full supportive and resuscitative measures, use of brain-shrinking drugs (hypertonic saline or mannitol), careful management of fever and blood glucose levels, and whether an individual under-goes decompressive craniectomy can affect recovery.

In case of a craniectomy, the bone flap (usually stored temporarily in a freezer) is replaced. Weeks later, additional reconstruction is done. As a patient regains mobility, a helmet is worn to protect the head during healing.

Decisions such as whether to proceed with more-aggressive measures, including surgery, should be based on a patient's prior stated wishes regarding living with a major impairment. If swelling isn't addressed, a fatal outcome is inevitable.

As I mentioned earlier in this book, small strokes can occur in crucial areas of the brain. When they do, an individual can look quite bad on admission. Because strokes in the brainstem are often small, the functional outcome for patients who have them is good. A stroke in the cerebellum or thalamus or in the occipital lobe can be quite disabling initially because it impairs stance, motility, vision and speech, but the outlook for functional recovery is quite good.

A clot in the basilar artery that causes a coma or locked-in syndrome poses a high risk of dying or not recovering function. That's why we try to remove such clots surgically when possible. In general, outcomes aren't very good for individuals who receive long-term care after large strokes in the brainstem, despite the best efforts at rehabilitation. Strokes in the occipital lobes also can be quite disabling, causing blindness.

Neurorehabilitation

In many cases of stroke, a patient's outcome is determined both by the brain's recovery potential and the results of rigorous neurorehabilitation. Neurorehabilitation doesn't necessarily increase the chances of improvement, but it can help an individual learn to adapt to the new handicap. How well comatose patients recover from major disabling symptoms varies, and it happens in very small steps.

Some neurologic impairments, such as difficulty speaking, may completely define an individual's disability, and resolving it improves daily functioning. Fortunately, we usually see substantial improvement in speech within the first two weeks after a stroke. The progress may continue for up to six months, after which it may reach a plateau. To a certain degree, speech therapy may help. Speech therapists are experts at finding new ways of communicating, and practicing their techniques can help promote recovery from a stroke.

Recovery of limb strength may take a long time, and many people experience persistent weakness and loss of function

LOCKED-IN SYNDROME

Locked-in syndrome is a rare neurologic condition in which there's complete paralysis of all voluntary muscles except for those that control movement of the eyes. Cognitive function is unaffected, and the individual is conscious and awake, but can't move or speak. Communication can only occur by way of eye movements and blinking, and with the help of sophisticated computers.

Some people with locked-in syndrome have written autobiographies about the frustration and loneliness of their new situations. Hope for further recovery was their major motivation.

It should be noted that a diagnosis of locked-in syndrome doesn't always mean a major deficit. Improvement may be seen in the first months and continue for years (albeit excruciatingly slowly). Many patients do improve to some degree, which may make communication easier. Improvement is more likely if, initially, they have more function than is typical with locked-in syndrome and, also, if they're younger. Surprisingly, in surveys of individuals with locked-in syndrome, the majority rated their quality of life as reasonable, considering the circumstances.

six months after a stroke. Better results are to be expected with the legs than the arms.

A brainstem stroke can cause other neurologic impairments, such as an inability to retain new memories (older memories are rarely lost), impaired vision or difficulty with balance when walking. For example, an individual who's had a stroke may not be able to see or feel one side of his or her body, making the world seem strange and unnatural. It's a major impediment to recovery. Physicians who aren't neurologists or experts in rehabilitation may not fully appreciate the difficulties a person faces when asked to exercise a limb in which there's no physical sensation, and in the person's view may as well have been amputated.

RECOVERY FROM A RUPTURED BRAIN ANEURYSM

A ruptured brain aneurysm is a neuro-critical emergency. Initially, the situation may look dire, but it may improve in a day or two after efforts to restore brain function. Approximately 1 in 5 individuals with a ruptured brain aneurysm who arrives at the hospital in a poor state may still have a good outcome without major disabling cognitive defects. About the same number will remain markedly impaired.

In the ICU, we often see patients improve rapidly after the first days of treatment but then start to plateau or even worsen. This is often a result of narrowing of the large brain arteries (vasospasm), which

reduces blood flow to the smaller arteries. Although expected, this major setback is hard on family members. The patient may be drowsy, sleepy, and very hard to awaken for days, but most get through it.

To raise blood pressure, more fluids and additional treatments are given, including medications to widen the blood vessels in the brain. The problem is, signs of reduced blood flow (ischemia) rarely appear until four days after a rupture, and there's considerable variation in their presentation. In most individuals, a change in brain function may first become apparent with a gradually decreased level of consciousness. Some may develop loss of speech or new agitation and disorientation.

We also know that 1 in 4 patients with a subarachnoid hemorrhage — bleeding in the space between the brain and the surrounding membrane — will undergo unexplained acute deterioration and then get better. Many improve after a neurosurgeon places a permanent drain.

Outcomes among individuals with subarachnoid hemorrhages often change in the long term. When these patients return for follow-up assessment after six months, they may still be experiencing considerable fatigue while performing day-to-day activities. But their mental clarity often is markedly improved. Studies also indicate that 1 in 3 people with a subarachnoid hemorrhage discharged to a nursing home in poor condition improve and are able to function independently within the first two years.

Approximately half the individuals who survive a ruptured aneurysm complain of difficulty with memory and other skills, which may lead to reduced quality of life. Roughly the same number have memory deficits that persist for more than a year after the event. In the second year after a ruptured aneurysm, some individuals may experience depression or anxiety.

All these complications affect quality of life and ability to resume roles with major responsibilities. Some individuals can no longer hold jobs. Despite gains in functional independence, many complain of cognitive impairment and dissatisfaction with their quality of life.

RECOVERY AFTER CARDIOPULMONARY RESUSCITATION

Years ago, predicting the prognosis of patients who received successful cardio-pulmonary resuscitation (CPR) was simpler. Today, the use of hypothermia and intravenous (IV) drugs to support CPR has significantly confounded the situation. For a true assessment, the medications must first be cleared by the kidneys and liver, and that may take time if those organs were temporarily or permanently damaged because the heart wasn't functioning.

Many studies examining CPR outcomes lack information regarding neurologic findings, sedation used, neuroimaging completed and how the individuals are functioning. This type of data is often crucial for assessing prognosis in these cases.

When patients improve, they typically do so rather quickly, as expected. This is why physicians often wait a few days to voice opinions about a patient's potential outcome. We've learned over the years that imposing a so-called "72-hour limit" may be problematic if the patient has received several drugs that need more time to clear from the body. Making a prognostic assessment of a poor outcome is only feasible if there are obvious signs of profound brainstem damage, which isn't common. Often, we give patients the benefit of the doubt; and indeed, that's appropriate in the absence of other major medical concerns.

People who awaken immediately following CPR may still experience acute states of confusion and long-term cognitive impairments. And they often have impaired short- and long-term memory. Some patients remain in a state of impaired awareness and interaction, with recovery heralded by periods of eye-opening. This is known as a vegetative state and is termed *persistent vegetative state* when it lasts for at least 30 days. Individuals who regain fragments of meaningful interaction and awareness of themselves or their environments are in a minimally conscious state.

Nearly half of cardiac arrest survivors successfully resuscitated and discharged from the hospital have cognitive and neuropsychiatric impairment. While long-term cognitive impairment is common in the critically ill, those who've experienced cardiac arrest have difficulty with attention, processing speed, executive function, memory and learning.

Patients treated with body temperature management — such as keeping the body's temperature at 36 C — have more than 50% better odds of experiencing no or only mild intellectual impairment, compared with those who don't undergo temperature control.

Recovery of memory typically occurs during the first three months. Regaining executive function — skills related to thinking, planning and self-control — can take 10 months or more. From 10% to 40% of patients experience seizures immediately after cardiac arrest, which may impact the prognosis. However, among individuals who have a seizure in the hospital after their hearts stop, the risk of developing later seizures is low — just 1% a year.

Basal ganglia injury may occur, which manifests as involuntary movements that resemble Parkinson's disease. It's effectively treated with medications. Irregular twitching or shocks (myoclonus) with movement may develop soon after the initial injury. These symptoms also respond well to medications. (In contrast to acute, generalized myoclonus, discussed in Chapter 5, myoclonus after CPR carries a more favorable outcome and resolves within months to years, even when initial treatment is aggressive.)

RECOVERY FROM BRAIN INFECTION

When treating infections in the brain, the aggressiveness of care generally determines a patient's outcome. Clearly, it's important to know if an individual has received aggressive treatment and is experiencing late complications, such as swelling (edema). In some instances, brain swelling can be effectively treated with brain-shrinking medications and high-dose corticosteroids in addition to antibiotics. Placement of a drain also may be necessary to reduce pressure.

A core principle is that recovery from a recent brain infection — no matter the cause — takes time. If early withdrawal of care is proposed for an individual who's still comatose several days after being treated with antibiotics or antiviral drugs, the outcome obviously will be worse. Physicians must resist the temptation to de-escalate care if a patient has plateaued for several weeks and consider it only if other major complications have occurred.

The outcome for patients with an infection-induced coma (bacterial or viral) depends on the level of unconsciousness when they're admitted and how soon they receive antibiotics or antiviral drugs. Time to antibiotic or antiviral treatment is a major determinant, and delay reduces the likelihood of a good outcome.

The most important factor for a good outcome with inflammation of the fluid and membranes surrounding the brain and spinal cord (bacterial meningitis) is absence of inflammation throughout the body triggered by infection-fighting chemicals (sepsis). Cause also matters; the odds of an unfavorable outcome are six times higher in patients infected with *Streptococcus pneumoniae* than in people infected with *Neisseria meningitidis*.

If an individual experiences a single brain abscess, prognosis often depends on whether the patient is a good surgical candidate. Most individuals with an isolated lesion are. Neurosurgery is more likely to produce favorable results if the abscess is superficial or located in the portion of the brain at the back of the skull (cerebellum). Antimicrobial therapy is often more appropriate for patients with deep-seated abscesses or abscesses involving small chambers or vesicles (multilocular), and among immuno-suppressed individuals with parasitic infections or with mold infections, such as aspergillosis.

Encephalitis-induced coma is associated with worse outcomes, largely because available treatments aren't very effective. The outcome of encephalitis varies, depending on a patient's age, duration of disease, and level of consciousness. Individuals younger than age 30 who remain largely alert have a higher chance of returning to their pre-infection level of functioning prior to their infection than do older patients with altered consciousness. A small proportion of patients will awaken, and an even smaller proportion will regain their independence.

There's no effective treatment for certain types of encephalitis. That's why the outcome often is poor. This includes rabies encephalitis, many of the fungal infections, and more recently, West Nile virus encephalitis. More invasive neurologic forms of encephalitis can cause loose and floppy limbs (flaccid paralysis) and marked changes in the brain and brainstem. Individuals requiring a mechanical ventilator may recover substantially over a period of several years.

RECOVERY FROM POISONING AND OVERDOSES

Many forms of poisoning and alcohol or drug intoxication may lead to permanent neurologic deficits.

Carbon monoxide poisoning

Early signs of carbon monoxide poisoning generally include personality changes, snapping at people, and outbursts of anxiety. Profound headache and coma also can occur with increased concentrations of carbon monoxide in the bloodstream.

Hyperbaric oxygen therapy is generally used to treat individuals experiencing symptoms. Patients who receive this treatment within 6 hours of carbon monoxide exposure generally have a better prognosis than those treated later. However, clinical trials haven't established whether the administration of hyperbaric oxygen therapy in patients with carbon monoxide poisoning reduces the incidence of adverse neurologic outcomes.

Alcohol poisoning

Ingestion of atypical alcohol — methanol found in commercial products such as windshield washer fluids, deicers, antifreeze, paints, wood stains, and glass cleaners — is very problematic and often fatal. Hard-to-detect inhalants, such as aerosols and dry-cleaning fluids, also contain brain-damaging substances that can be fatal. Treatment generally involves use of an antidote, and dialysis is often recommended.

Overdoses of typical alcohols, such as beer, wine and hard liquor, generally involves supportive care while the body rids itself of the alcohol.

Drug overdoses

Unfortunately, coma resulting from drug abuse has significantly increased due to the opioid epidemic. An opioid overdose, which happens most often through heroin injection or use of oxycodone for chronic pain management, can cause permanent brain injury.

Heroin users may remain comatose for weeks and MRI scans will reveal dramatic brain changes. Despite the changes, these individuals may still awaken, and their cognition may substantially improve. There may be some long-term complications, certainly with repeated overdoses.

When examining a patient whose coma was caused by a drug overdose, there generally are two extremely important determinations a neurologist will make: 1) whether the injury is permanent; and 2) whether continuous EEG monitoring is needed to identify and manage ongoing seizures.

Active heroin or oxycodone users potentially can survive an overdose if naloxone is administered by a bystander. This opioid overdose reversal has been shown in naloxone programs. It's a simple, yet important observation. Studies also have found that the risk of heroin overdose and death increases in the first 12 months after addiction therapy is discontinued and the first two weeks after a user is released from incarceration. Therefore, an argument can be made for providing patients with take-home naloxone to prevent these lethal events.

RECOVERY FROM CONTINUED SEIZURES

An individual's outcome after experiencing a seizure depends on the type of seizure and what provoked it. Among individuals with epilepsy, causes of the seizures are quite diverse, and in many people, a cause can be found. In people who experience an epileptic episode, the treatment the individual receives may affect his or her outcome. Time to treatment of epilepsy matters, but often treatment is delayed or may be inappropriate. Treatment of prolonged seizures is complex and generally involves many intravenous drugs.

Predicting prognosis in patients with epilepsy is incredibly hard because many of them have surprisingly good outcomes. Some individuals manage to pull themselves out of a seizure, and there are many examples of good outcomes among individuals who initially didn't respond well to treatment.

Some studies have suggested that an hour or more of untreated, continuous twitching may indicate a poor outcome, but multiple other reports have not supported this. Encephalitis often is associated with a high proportion of uncontrolled seizures, and survivors have a substantial risk of long-term seizures. The outcome after a seizure episode also is poor if the underlying disorder is a terminal illness, such as recurrence of a brain tumor, and most certainly if an individual has a rapidly worsening genetic metabolic disorder.

The outcome often is much different in individuals who have prolonged seizures in rapid succession. Typically, most patients with a flurry of seizures do just fine, assuming there's no other major neurologic illness. But individuals who are comatose and have uncontrolled seizures that don't respond to multiple drugs or who experience a recurrence every time intravenous medications are reduced often don't do well.

RECOVERY FROM PROLONGED COMA

As I've mentioned previously, we see very few patients in vegetative states, either because such a state is rare or because families make the decision not to prolong life in keeping with their loved ones' wishes.

There's some truth in saying that people in vegetative states never recover because they're never given the opportunity to recover. Based on a patient's previously expressed wishes, the family and health care team decide not to treat complica-

tions, and the individual dies. However, by addressing every serious complication, administering superb nursing care, and undergoing full resuscitative measures, the individual in a vegetative state may have a small chance of some type of recovery.

For years, the general thinking in the medical community has been that people who are in vegetative states for more than three months after a coma that wasn't trauma related won't regain substantial awareness. We draw a similar conclusion about individuals who've been comatose more than a year after traumatic brain injuries. However, recent reports suggest that some individuals regain minimal consciousness (meaning more awareness) after long periods in a comatose state.

When coma is prolonged, the likelihood of recovery decreases over a relatively short time, generally because the individuals develop complications, many of them life-threatening from being confined to a bed. However, prolonged survival can be achieved with meticulous care and aggressive medical intervention when a complication develops. Of course, this level of care is extremely expensive, and this isn't a perfect world in which money is no object.

There are several examples of individuals in vegetative states who've been kept alive for decades. In these cases, do we hold on to the slim hope that an individual may recover? I don't know. When I look at a horrific brain scan that shows that large parts of a patient's brain have turned into fluid and cysts, making it neurologically impossible for that person to recover, I ask myself why we continue to treat every possible complication.

Late recoveries following a persistent vegetative state have been described, one of which occurred in an individual seven years after brain injury stemming from a heart attack and CPR. However, all the patients who reportedly have "recovered" have remained in severely disabled states, fully dependent on care, confined to a bed or wheelchair, fed through a feeding tube, and unable to control their bladders or bowels. Their responses are inconsistent and not reproducible, and it's questionable whether the individuals' humanity and dignity have been preserved.

Factors that may predict recovery from a prolonged persistent vegetative state haven't been identified. Do studies suggest the possibility of late recovery from prolonged coma, or were the patients described in these cases simply misdiagnosed? It's hard to tell, because so few individuals in vegetative states survive more than a year or two.

I should refute one more misunderstanding, which is that awakening leads to more distress due to despair and frustration as the individual becomes aware of his or her disabilities. There's little evidence that this is true, and it hasn't been noted by most rehabilitation physicians.

A LONG JOURNEY

Caretakers and family members should be prepared for periods of one step forward, two steps back. Simple things they used to take for granted now seem unreachable. Problems that existed before a loved one's brain injury now seem less important.

In older individuals, general physical frailty is a huge issue. Other medical issues or social and family circumstances also may intervene, leading to a change in priorities. It's never one size fits all, and different approaches may be needed for different individuals. Some family members cope with the situation by denying or disavowing what's happening, making it difficult to communicate openly with health care staff.

Some individuals may experience a discrete decline in their ability to remember, have a tendency to misplace things, need to rely on notes and reminders, repeat questions, and lose track of dates, but they can still live independently with a loved one or spouse. Still, long-term care, in-home rehabilitation, home-based educational interventions, and caregiver support may all be necessary to keep a loved one out of a hospital or nursing facility.

Setting priorities for the care of a patient who awakens from a coma is important. According to Leslie Scheunemann, M.D., a geriatric medicine specialist and intensive care physician, several aspects are crucial (see page 86).

For many individuals, the only approach is to make do with the function they have. Neurologic disability after coma recovery is difficult to describe and to judge in the first weeks following an injury. The onus is on an experienced neurologist to explain what neurologic disability means for day-to-day living. How the individual was functioning before the traumatic event should also be considered, and we should allow this the information to guide our decisions as well.

However, rarely do patients make a complete recovery after a major brain injury. The extent of the recovery generally has more to do with an individual's adaptability than with a true return of function, but the results can still be very good.

Understand that rehabilitation can't achieve the impossible goal of walking out of a center as if nothing happened. It may not speed recovery, but it definitely plays a major role in a person's ability to adapt. Clearly, the brain can adapt, but often on its own schedule.

Coma survivors often are encouraged to "learn to live with" their disability, but I think that's an oversimplification. What's required is a change in mindset. Priorities, too, must change. What used to be important may have to wait for another day or not be considered at all. Determination and stamina are hard to measure, but individuals who can stay focused progress better after awakening from their comas.

Poor health, such as heart and lung disease, diabetes and obesity, as well as severe depression, may hamper recovery, and, unfortunately, these can't be easily reversed.

PRIORITIES FOR PATIENTS ONCE THEY LEAVE THE ICU

- Feeling safe (knowing what to do when something happens)
- Being comfortable (no disabling pain)
- Mobility (ability to sit, stand, walk, climb stairs)
- Being able to provide self-care (toileting, bathing, grooming)
- Being able to resume leisure activities
- Being able to socialize with friends and family
- Having personal dignity (feeling respected)
- Well-being of family members (OK and not stressed out)
- Going home (main goal)
- Getting better physically (seeing progress)
- Getting better psychologically (not down and out)
- Being able to move on (getting over it)

Based on Scheunemann L., et al. *Annals of the American Thoracic Society.* 2020;17: 221.

AND FINALLY

Rehabilitation has allowed many survivors of major brain injuries to return to their previous lives — or as close as possible. Good outcomes often stem from a multidisciplinary team of experts in occupational and speech therapy, neuropsychology, and social work who evaluate a patient's goals and achievements on a weekly basis. This type of support system is absolutely essential while an individual is going through various stages of recovery.

This chapter provides a fairly optimistic view of potential outcomes after awakening from being comatose. It's a reminder that a good outcome is very possible, even among individuals who arrive at hospitals in severe states.

There will always be people who defy all odds. Most often, these tend to be young individuals who often undergo months of care and rehabilitation. I've even witnessed good outcomes in patients with unrelenting seizures who could only be kept in check with continued use of anti-epileptic medications, but who were young and otherwise healthy. Yet we still must be cautious and not become overly optimistic in anticipating prognosis, even among young individuals.

When is recovery not likely to happen?

5

A CONVERSATION

Physician: Your husband is at a point where we need to step back and consider what he's achieved.

Family: We're very worried. It doesn't seem like he's improved.

Physician: I'm sorry, but I have the unfortunate responsibility of telling people things they'd rather not hear. Regarding your husband, I don't believe that he will recover to a degree that we'd all feel is acceptable.

Family: Please be frank with us about his condition. Tell us what decisions we may need to make.

Neurologists often see patients who have devastating neurologic injuries and are not expected to improve, or who may even get worse. It's an uncomfortable situation, but one we take very seriously. Only after we've observed a patient for a sufficient time, performed important clinical assessments and have test results that definitively point toward a bad outcome do we broach the subject of lack of recovery with family.

At times such as these, doctors need to call it as they see it. Deliberate exaggeration has no role in any profession and certainly not in a medical environment. Equally, truth doesn't come in small steps or after detours. Family members want to know and understand, and they should be reassured that no physician takes these conversations lightly.

We don't view a poor outcome as a personal defeat but more as a fact of nature, despite our flaws and the ever-present unpredictability of a patient's time in the hospital. Making a well-informed assessment of what the coming weeks and months will bring for an individual is an essential part of practicing medicine. We don't take hope away, but we need to be realistic. Avoiding the prognosis, always presenting the bright side, and using euphemisms and equivocation are what Nicholas Christakis, in his book *Death Foretold*, calls the ritualization of optimism.

One fact about brain injury is indisputable: What's gone is gone. But that doesn't mean recovery is impossible. Are other parts of the brain taking over? Are parts of the brain simply stunned and getting ready to function again? Do we just need to await regrowth with new connections? Who has a chance and who doesn't? How can we tell? Those questions we address in Chapter 4. In this chapter, I try to explain what defines a poor outcome and why we can predict such an outcome with certainty in some situations.

When doctors discuss a patient's outcome, we never forget we could be wrong and sometimes very wrong. I accept unpredictability with brain injuries and acknowledge that I sometimes might have to reconsider the diagnosis. I'm mindful of situations that can fool us and prompt an incorrect outcome assessment. Sometimes a patient's recovery will take longer than expected, and doctors need to postpone important decisions and step back.

This chapter focuses on individuals who are not changing for the better and the consequences of that interpretation. Some circumstances that lead to coma are so rare that it's impossible to predict the outcome among patients who experience them. Environmental injuries such as electrocution and lightning strikes are examples. When we see them, we can't rely on prior examples and other accounts in the medical literature.

When an individual is found unconscious without clues about the circumstances that caused it, predicting outcome is difficult. The best approach is repeated clinical examination, using MRI to find or exclude injury, and then interpreting the severity of injury by comparing it to other, similar situations.

SOME NUMBERS AND PERCENTAGES

Neurologists often work differently from other specialists. When we encounter comatose patients whom we consider to be in bad situations, we're seeing them at the most severe stage of their illness. Reliably predicting an outcome isn't possible for many of these individuals, and we have to base our clinical judgment on test results.

Often, this means neurologic examinations in the intensive care unit (ICU) over time — daily, weekly and sometimes monthly after a patient is transferred to a general floor. We always want to give an individual a fighting chance to improve, but on the other hand, in some situations, that's extraordinarily unlikely. It's also not possible to estimate a patient's odds of recovery using percentages, although some people want us to do that. That's because even if the chances of recovery are less than 1%, some patients will still jump through all the hoops and make a recovery. We simply have no way to identify them.

Medicine is full of elusive numbers, and all the percentages can be dizzying. Number-based decision-making is significant and taxing. Moreover, numbers don't appear in a vacuum, and percentages have a so-called range, also known as the 95% confidence interval (CI). The 95% CI is a range of values for which we can be 95% confident that they reflect the true value of the population. Bear with me here.

For example, let's assume studies looking at the chance of recovery for certain causes of coma show that 3% will recover. The 95% CI of that number is between 0%

and 10%. That means there is still a 5% chance that recovery could be greater than 10%. Some could argue this isn't certain enough. We often must hear this a few times to understand it properly. Even then, some family members may still be optimistic despite hearing the physician express serious doubt.

Clearly, numbers or graphs are difficult for many of us to grasp or see in a larger context. Studies have found that expressing numbers in different ways — such as saying 1 in 25 or 4% — makes a difference in how outcome is perceived. One in 25 is better understood than the abstract 4%. This isn't a trivial matter. The images below are examples of what 4% looks like in graphic form and how different it may seem when presented in other ways.

You may have heard the phrase "reasonable medical certainty." What does that mean? In his classic article on reasonable medical certainty, psychiatrist Jonas R.

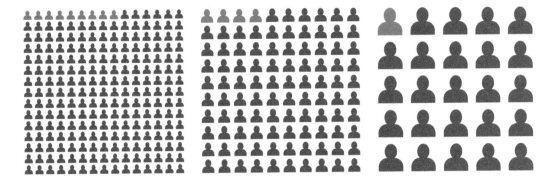

This graphic displays different ways of showing and interpreting percentages. Most people perceive the graph on the right (1 in 25 people) as showing a greater chance of a poor outcome than is displayed by the other graphs. But they're all the same: 1 in 25, 9 in 225 and 4 in 100 all equate to 4%.

Rappeport said, "There's no simple answer. Reasonable medical certainty is not what I thought it was. It's neither reasonable nor certain. It may be a probability, but then it's quite possible it's a possibility."

WHEN NOTHING CAN BE DONE

Within the range of poor outcomes, there are patients whose situations are truly hopeless (see the shaded box below). This determination is usually based on clear abnormalities on a CT scan and continued poor results on neurological examinations after aggressive and continued therapy. Sometimes, we reach this determination after we've performed last-resort brain surgery with absolutely no change afterward.

When we first see a patient, we may know that the outcome is likely to be poor despite our efforts, but providing options to patients and families makes us feel a lot better. It may be futile and perhaps even exasperating, but it's human nature to leave no stone unturned, so we can honestly say we tried everything. We can never say that the chance of recovery is poor until we've tried everything — within reason.

That said, there's a limit to what can be done, and we don't necessarily do everything when it makes no sense. Brain surgery, for example, shouldn't be offered if a patient's brain is terribly damaged. We know that the outcome will be poor. Damage from some brain injuries is so overwhelmingly catastrophic that nothing can be done.

In addition, we've learned over many years that brainstem injuries are often very significant. We discover significant injuries by testing the brainstem for the absence or failure of common reflexes.

INDICATIONS THAT TREATMENT IS FUTILE AND A POOR OUTCOME IS LIKELY

- Massive brain swelling and brainstem injury
- Major stroke in the brainstem (often a destructive bleed)
- Inability to remove a blood clot in the basilar artery that provides blood to the brainstem
- Seizures and constant irregular twitching (myoclonus) in the face, arms and legs in an unresponsive patient after cardiac arrest
- Gunshot wound to the head that crosses both sides of the brain
- Other conditions that make improvement doubtful (end-stage cancer, progressive liver and kidney failure, shock, very poor health before the event that led to coma)

What we do know, however, is that long waiting times don't necessarily lead to full recovery. Although most comatose patients do awaken, it doesn't mean they awaken wholly restored.

Sometimes, a patient may show initial signs of improvement but then have a complication such as a major infection or we detect something unexpected, such as cancer that's spread to the brain from elsewhere in the body. That's why with each person we must look at the bigger picture. Sometimes we have to consider the functioning of other organs and whether a brain injury on top of an already marginal preexisting medical state will make recovery impossible.

Let's review those conditions that experience tells us are most likely to lead to a poor outcome in which a patient is unlikely to improve.

Traumatic brain injury

Predicting how an individual with a brain injury from trauma is likely to fare can be difficult. That's because these individuals tend to be younger, and they have resilient brains. As a result, they may improve, often to a very surprising extent.

Rarely do physicians come to a definitive conclusion that care is futile unless the person is close to losing all brain function. For example, a penetrating injury, such as from a gunshot, in which an object has traversed both parts of the brain can be considered unsalvageable, and this is often evident when the person is first examined.

Over the years, I've seen individuals in very poor condition, including some with brainstem injuries, crawl out of a deep pit and make gradual improvements. Young patients who were basically in a vegetative state and transferred from the ICU to a nursing home have walked into our unit years later to thank the health care staff.

Recovery may take longer when surgery is required to remove bruised tissue and relieve pressure or a major blood clot on the brain after a traumatic brain injury. Even when such a procedure succeeds, improvement still can take several weeks. The recovery needle may move in the wrong direction if the patient displays ominous signs, such as pupils that don't respond to light or spasms in the arms and legs. Still, these aren't unequivocal indicators of a hopeless prognosis in every case.

While many comatose patients recover, we know from the very start in others, the outcome is likely to be poor. A major determinant is sustained, increased intracranial pressure. This typically happens in individuals with trauma to the brainstem and loss of many brainstem reflexes. In anyone with traumatic brain injury, the presence of storming — spells of profuse sweating, fever, stiffening up, jaw clenching and teeth grinding — indicates a very severe brain injury.

Whether aggressive, early treatment affects outcome in such cases is unknown. I've rarely seen any of these patients make a perfectly good recovery. Most of them end up in nursing homes and don't make enough progress to qualify for admission to a rehabilitation center.

When examination and test results are consistently poor, we often conclude that rescue surgery isn't an option. Rising pressure in the brain due to massive swelling usually can't be reversed unless the patient is young, generally younger than age 40. Most individuals older than age 80 can't tolerate trauma to the brain well, and a freak fall may completely change the outlook, even if they previously functioned at a high level.

Poor outcomes after traumatic brain injury are expected in older individuals in a sustained coma, as well as in younger individuals who have lost many brainstem reflexes.

Another influencing factor regarding whether to continue treatment is devastating findings on MRI, particularly if prolonged lack of oxygen caused brain damage. In fact, many individuals who do poorly after a major traumatic brain injury had a difficult and prolonged resuscitation, which may be evident on an MRI.

Stroke

As explained in Chapter 2, ischemic stroke halts blood flow to a part of the brain. Blood flow can also be impaired due to hemorrhagic stroke, which causes bleeding into the brain. An ischemic stroke cuts off blood flow, whereas a hemorrhagic stroke allows too much blood into the brain.

Acute ischemic or even hemorrhagic stroke doesn't always cause loss of consciousness. After a stroke, individuals often are alert, although many don't fully realize what has happened to them. Most acute strokes occur in small arteries or involve a part of the brain that barely affects structures governing alertness and awareness. Declining responsiveness in an individual who's had a stroke may have another cause, such as the effects of sedative drugs administered during transport, a laboratory abnormality such as a rapid spike in blood sugar, or a seizure.

A stroke-induced coma signals a very serious problem. Coma after a stroke usually, but not always, indicates large areas of destruction, such as a great deal of bleeding in the brain. A stroke in the brainstem due to a clot in the basilar artery is another common cause of initially unexplained coma. Even a small area of damage in the brainstem may interrupt arousal mechanisms.

Hemorrhagic stroke

When a coma is due to severe bleeding (a large hemorrhage), the result is a shift in volume and pressure on other structures. Conventional wisdom once was that bleeding in the brain would resolve quickly, but we now know that bleeding can continue and have a snow-ball effect.

Prognosis in an individual with a deteriorating hemorrhagic stroke generally depends on whether it is possible to remove the clot causing the bleeding and how soon surgery can take place. Location of the clot is another factor. Many clots lodge deep in the brain and can only be reached by cutting into healthy surrounding tissue, which neurosurgeons are very reluctant to do. Moreover, clinical trials have shown that the outcome may be worse when deep clots are removed. Other therapies, such as using a catheter to suck out the clot, have been tried, but often the clot returns. Clotting medications may stop bleeding in the brain, but they may cause clots in other arteries, creating a worse problem.

Bleeding in the brainstem and in the cerebellum in the back of the head is much less common but very dramatic. Patients may arrive in the emergency room in a deep coma or spiral downward in a matter of hours. Bleeding in the brainstem that produces coma often is so severe that we don't expect any improvement; it's one of the worst possible strokes. However, the outcome can be quite good if the cause is blood in the cerebellum that's pressing on the brainstem and the blood clot can be removed. That's why these patients need to be seen by a neurosurgeon right away.

Ischemic stroke

The effects of a coma from ischemic stroke are similar. A tissue shift in the brain due to swelling must be treated by removing part of the skull to allow for swelling outside the skull (decompression). If such surgery isn't possible, the outcome often is poor. While decompression often can positively influence outcome in younger individuals, it's of less benefit to individuals older than age 60.

Strokes in the thalamus near the center of the brain (see Chapter 1) immediately alter consciousness, but patients may awaken, often after a period of markedly fluctuating alertness. An acute clot in the basilar artery in the brainstem is devastating, but if CT scan results are normal, quickly removing the clot with a catheter can be very successful. There's a risk, however, that the artery may not open during the procedure. If that happens, the patient won't recover function.

Aneurysm

Predicting outcome in an individual with a ruptured aneurysm is complex and difficult. If a drain is placed or the clot is removed from the brain soon after the rupture, the patient may improve rapidly within hours after the procedure. But if most brainstem reflexes remain lost after such interventions, recovery is rare. Many patients with brain aneurysms have large ventricles filled with blood, and many have already experienced a re-bleed, which is a critical factor in potential outcome.

Other major factors that point to poorer outcomes are spasm in an artery and an inability to control it effectively with medication. As with other causes of coma, age greatly influences outcome, and in individuals older than age 80, survival that includes meaningful functioning is uncommon.

Infections

Infection of the lining of the brain (meningitis) and infection of brain tissues (encephalitis) can be treated with antibiotics, antiviral drugs or medications such as corticosteroids that suppress the immune system. Other therapies also are very helpful.

Patients with meningitis or encephalitis who are comatose are obviously in a worse state, but many will improve, often over a matter of weeks and, sometimes, within days. I've seen barely responsive patients with meningitis improve dramatically after receiving the right antibiotics. However, if an infection in the arteries leading to the brain or clots in the brain's venous system cause strokes, a good outcome becomes significantly less likely.

Some brain infections, such as rabies encephalitis, are so devastating that there's no chance of a good outcome. Although rabies is very uncommon in western countries, it has a nearly 100% mortality rate. There's also no effective treatment for many fungal infections of the brain or for West Nile virus encephalitis, and therefore, outcome is poor. In individuals with suppressed immune systems, these infections can be particularly devastating.

Some patients with meningitis recover fully, but more invasive neurologic forms can cause marked changes in many parts of the brain. In general, 20% of patients with West Nile virus encephalitis die, and death is much more likely in older adults. The prognosis may be poor for younger patients who need mechanical ventilation, but some may recover substantially over a period of several years.

Herpes simplex encephalitis is a common infection that also can cause significant injury to the brain. Most patients do awaken, but they may have markedly impaired memory and speech.

The encephalitis with the best overall outcome is so-called autoimmune encephalitis. In this condition, the immune system attacks the brain or certain parts of it for an unknown reason. This can cause seizures and coma. Once the seizures are controlled, there's a chance for improvement provided the individual's immune system is muted and held in check. Sometimes autoimmune encephalitis is due to undetected cancer. In those cases, a good outcome also involves identifying and treating the cancer.

Autoimmune encephalitis is seen mainly in younger patients, and thus, outcomes tend to be better than for encephalitis that develops in older individuals.

Brain abscesses

Pus that collects in the brain from an infection is called a brain abscess. The outcome of a single brain abscess is dependent on whether a patient is a good surgical candidate. Neurosurgery often is considered if an abscess isn't deep (superficial) or located in the cerebellum. Antibiotics are more appropriate than surgery in deep-seated abscesses or if an individual has several abscesses. They're also preferable for patients with suppressed immune systems and small, widespread abscesses.

The chances for recovery are poor if the patient is comatose before an abscess is treated and, particularly, if the abscess has ruptured into brain ventricles. When that happens, a severe meningitis will cause a rapid decline and, often, death. Multiple brain abscesses are a concern because their entry into the brain's ventricles allows deep spread of the infection and generally results in a poor outcome.

Deaths from brain abscesses are less likely than they once were because abscesses can be detected earlier with MRI and, therefore, treated more quickly. Neurosurgeons often place a catheter into the cavity to drain the pus. Other treatments include prescribing antibiotics or antifungal medications or using a catheter and medication in combination. However, antibiotics don't always help in these cases.

Inadequate oxygen to the brain

Cardiac arrest means no effective contraction of the heart muscle and no blood flow to the brain, which leads to sudden loss of consciousness. Halted blood flow injures the brain because it deprives the brain's neurons of oxygen, which they need to function. The longer this continues, the worse the outcome.

Next to having an emergency responder on the spot when a heart attack occurs, the best hope is a proactive bystander who knows how to do CPR. If the chest compressions aren't fast and deep enough and timed with mouth-to-mouth resuscitation, the effort may be inadequate. The outcome of cardiac arrest is also much worse when no one is available to start chest compressions immediately.

FACTS ABOUT RESUSCITATION AFTER CARDIAC ARREST

- 1 in 4 patients survives an in-hospital cardiac arrest.
- 1 in 2 patients survives after having a fibrillating and not-pumping heart (ventricular fibrillation) shocked into rhythm.
- 1 in 10 patients with a flatlined heart (asystole) survives more than one year.
- 2 of 3 patients who awaken, interact with their surroundings, and make it home have acceptable neurologic outcomes (some may have mental difficulties but are independent).

We don't know how long the brain can tolerate absent or markedly diminished blood flow. Even with the best resuscitation efforts, the blood pushed forward to the brain is just a fraction of what it should be. The extent of injury, however, often is variable. Bad outcomes can occur after short resuscitations and good outcomes after long ones.

Once the heart starts beating again and there's subsequent return of spontaneous circulation through the body and good blood pressure, a person's brain can potentially resume its function. The window for this to happen, however, is small. The abrupt cessation of blood flow virtually stops the brain's complex machinery. Calcium floods into brain cells leading to very severe damage.

Additional injury also can occur when circulation is restored and blood flows back into damaged areas. The resumption of blood flow can activate an inflammatory-stress response, damaging the blood-brain barrier and causing additional fluid to leak into the brain, further exacerbating cerebral swelling. Many of these harmful pathways are active for hours to days after circulation has been restored.

Patients whose hearts have stopped and been restarted may remain in a coma and not awaken even after steps to reduce swelling. A CT scan of the brain may show early brain swelling, which occurs if large parts of the cortex and deeper structures are involved. The swelling may also cause brain waves on an electroencephalogram (EEG) to flatten and not change when the patient is touched (lost reactivity). MRI is better for localizing and classifying the injury, but even MRI can produce repeatedly normal results in individuals who never awaken. As MRI technology and image resolution continue to improve, we may gain an understanding about why this occurs.

Among individuals resuscitated after cardiac arrest, the most helpful test for evaluating brain activity is a recording of somatosensory-evoked potentials (SSEP). This test evaluates the integrity of the pathways in a nerve that begins in an arm and extends into the spinal cord and up to the brainstem before ending in the cerebral cortex. Each structure along the way gives off a waveform after the nerve is shocked over 100 times. The absence of the N20 waveform in the cortex is always associated with a very poor outcome and, often, prolonged coma. Absence of N20s may be an even better predictor of poor outcome than a bedside neurological examination. However, relying on a test that shows absence of something is problematic because the same result could occur if the test was done incorrectly or it was performed correctly but the patient moved too much.

Widespread implementation of SSEPs truly requires advanced neurophysiologic training and experienced interpretation. This type of expertise often is only available in large medical centers. Many hospitals don't offer this potentially very useful test.

What all of this means is that most of the time we are fully reliant on a neurologic examination. The brainstem is usually unaffected by lack of oxygen, but when pupil reflexes are absent or an individual has only primitive responses such as posturing, indications of improvement must begin very quickly (generally within days) if the patient is going to have any chance of recovery.

Several studies have shown particularly poor outcomes in patients who experience ongoing seizures or muscle jerks (myoclonus). When these symptoms occur, we can anticipate a prolonged coma, and patients may never fully awaken. Often, the best that we can hope for is a minimally conscious state, in which individuals opens their eyes and look about at times but aren't clearly aware of and can't engage with their surroundings.

We've learned that improvement is most often seen in the first 3 to 7 days after a person becomes comatose. After that time, the chances become slimmer, although some patients do improve after longer periods of coma. When we place tracheostomy and gastrostomy tubes needed to improve long-term care, this is the juncture when we review an individual's history and test results and carefully consider which path to recommend to loved ones.

Often, neurologists can't reliably predict the outcome of brain injury after cardiac arrest, and it's become even more complicated recently because methods used to cool patients delay the clearance of drugs from their bodies for days and sometimes weeks.

However, there's no question that an individual's situation is dire if we see major damage on MRI, an SSEP test shows that signals from nerves aren't reaching the brain's cortex, and the person is experiencing seizures or continuous muscle twitching in the face, belly, arms and legs. Only rarely have I seen patients in this condition awaken from a coma and then improve, and none of them attained a quality of life that most people would consider acceptable. Continuation of intensive care for these patients often means 24-hour nursing care.

In addition, cardiac arrest often occurs in at-risk individuals with a history of heart failure or lung disease. This bigger picture often drives decision-making. We need to review the multitude of serious medical conditions that a patient has and their ramifications. We can't look at one organ system alone.

I should emphasize one more important fact. Brain damage can potentially occur if blood flow is adequate but there's not enough oxygen in the blood. This is very uncommon and requires a severe dip in oxygen levels. Very low oxygen alone occurs in patients who have acute severe lung disease. (We've all seen plenty of that during the SARS-CoV-2 pandemic.) These patients may take longer to recover, but if they have no other complications, their recovery is often truly remarkable. The worst injury is one that results from both no blood flow and lack of oxygen to the brain. That's far worse than any trauma, infection or stroke. The brain can't tolerate oxygen deprivation for more than a minute.

TALKING TO THE FAMILY

Once the medical team has assessed a comatose patient's condition, family members need to be informed about what to expect. Some will opt to continue life support, holding on to the remote possibility of improvement. We honor that, but only after repeated discussions emphasizing that they must be prepared for an extremely frustrating experience.

After viewing brain scans and hearing the results of medical assessments, other families accept the prognosis and confer among themselves about what their loved ones would have preferred. Again, it should be emphasized that none of these decisions is ours to make. Decisions should be based on the family's best assessment of how the patient would have wanted to live life.

A living will or advance health care directive can help in making decisions. Sometimes, a patient may have had prior conversations with close relatives about end-of-life concerns and expressed personal wishes. All of these factors should be taken into consideration in determining what an individual would want. It's cruel to ignore someone's stated wishes if those wishes are known. It's even worse if a patient is aware of a deficit and is powerless to change anything and faces a life of medical complications.

Surveys of people in the U.S. indicate that most people want to respect a loved one's wishes and minimize suffering. However, families can't always do so. In about 25% of cases, not all family members are in agreement as to whether care should be prolonged or stopped. Studies also indicate that concerns about a doctor's prognosis sometimes can keep families from following a loved one's wishes. In at least one survey, surprisingly, 1 in 3 families doubted the accuracy of the prognosis given to a loved one.

Families typically want physicians to tell them what to expect, but sometimes opinions differ and can't be reconciled. Family members may lose confidence in a physician who seems uncertain. Others believe that physicians will never be able to predict anything with the certainty that they'd like. Discussions with family members may turn sour if a health care provider is too confrontational or disrespectful or if the provider takes away all hope. Families often expect physicians to speak positively and provide hope for a good recovery, but doing so isn't always possible.

Cultural differences, too, may impact communication. Sometimes, family members suspect cultural bias or discrimination from health care staff. Some distrust may relate to conflicts within the family structure, many of which are unknown to the physician treating the patient. Far more often, health care staff is concerned about a family's interpersonal relationships when anger in the family escalates. (See Chapter 10 for further discussion and explanation.)

My underlying premise is that it doesn't make much sense to escalate care, be heroic or choose last-resort measures in a patient with a basically unrecoverable

LEVELS OF ICU CARE

This chart shows levels of care in an intensive care unit (ICU) and depicts reasonable approaches to care, depending on the patient's circumstances.

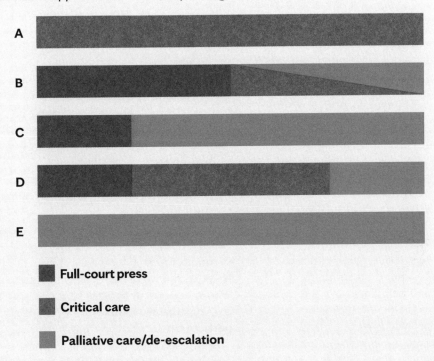

■ Full-court press

■ Critical care

■ Palliative care/de-escalation

A. Patient with unlimited continued critical care. Full benefit of care and a potentially good outcome is rightly anticipated.

B. Aggressive resuscitation with gradual limited critical care and gradual increasing de-escalation. This pathway is considered when, after resuscitation, the patient continues to decline and the function of other organs dwindles.

C. Aggressive resuscitation is attempted but is rapidly followed by symptom relief (palliative care) when the heroic action was to no avail.

D. Aggressive resuscitation followed by continued critical care, but a major complication occurs and the decision is made to provide palliative care only.

E. Poor outcome with no benefit already evident on admission and no treatment other than comfort measures.

disorder. Generally, it's important for families to understand the bigger picture and for health care providers and families to work together to resolve any concerns.

The chart on page 101 summarizes different treatment routes for patients who are comatose. Every individual we see eventually falls into one of these categories.

Our general principle is to postpone final decisions until after a period of maximal care, unless the tragedy that befell an individual was devastating from the very start. First, we apply short-term aggressive care ("full-court press") with gradual de-escalation if there's no change in a patient's neurologic condition. In these situations, we see the role of palliative care (treating symptoms, reducing discomfort and pain) increase in inverse proportion to the de-escalation of critical care. The more we let go of critical care, the more we need to consider appropriate comfort care.

The second approach is a more abrupt transition. The decision reached is to give any feasible medical or surgical option one more try, and if the treatment is unsuccessful, quickly abandon critical care. In the third approach, aggressive care with all resuscitative measures is followed by continued critical care. But when a major, unexpected complication occurs, the decision is made to provide only palliative care.

Finally, palliative care is initiated immediately in patients with a very poor prognosis; they aren't transferred back to ICUs and are given only peace, quiet and comfort.

It's important for family members to understand that predicting outcome is complex and flawed. On occasion, I've seen patients do reasonably well after being sent to a hospice. We've seen unexpected awakenings and, frankly, family claims of a miracle. Some individuals defy all odds and don't fit algorithms. This doesn't absolve health care professionals from their moral obligation to discuss their best assessment of a patient's condition and make decisions about which level of care seems appropriate.

Family members sometimes want a second opinion, which may or may not be helpful, and we usually ask colleagues who specialize in palliative care to participate. Decisions can be revisited, particularly if there are questions or if an individual's condition hasn't been correctly understood. Guilt is a strong emotion, but we always need to work from the basic premise that we're making decisions for the patient and that none of those decisions is our own. We often know what a patient wants.

AND FINALLY

What comes next for family members after I visit with them and tell them their loved one is unlikely to recover is heartbreaking. I've seen it again and again. They must explain to other family members who weren't present during our conversation what was said and discuss with them what to do next. These are very emotional conversations. Additional phone calls follow until all family members agree that their loved one has suffered enough, would never want to go on like this, and this is the end.

This point generally marks the beginning of remembrance, recalling the many good times that preceded the current situation. It's important for family members to accept that their loved one will be with them every day, in some fashion or another, and they will find themselves reflecting often on wonderful times spent together.

What is palliation, or comfort care?

6

A CONVERSATION

Physician: Let's talk about your father's condition and his lack of progress. His complications have been treated successfully, but neurologically, there are no signs of improvement.

Family: We noticed that, too, and we're worried.

Physician: I want to be upfront with you. May I share my concerns?

Family: We know what you're going to say.

Physician: I'm sorry, but we've run out of options. It's very likely that your father won't get better, and we strongly suspect that he'll remain in this state for the rest of his life. He won't be going home.

Family: We don't think going to a nursing home is an option. Being bedridden and tube-fed would be unacceptable to him. He'd be very mad at us if we let this continue. I suppose this means then that we should let him go.

Physician: If we all feel that those are his wishes, let's talk about how we can support him in this transition.

We've come to perhaps the most emotionally charged chapter of this book — the decision to withhold aggressive, active medical intervention and provide only comfort care for a loved one. There are several words for this stage of care at the end of life — comfort care, palliative care, palliation, suspending life-sustaining treatment — and all are similar in meaning. At this point, we've done all we can, and there are no other options, within reason.

A DELICATE TOPIC

The decision to seek comfort care is made when family and the medical team have concluded, without any doubt, that a patient has reached the very final stage. Anything we could do would be clinically inappropriate and not in the best interest of the individual. And maintaining the current level of critical care could cause medically unjustifiable harm.

At this juncture, the nature of care changes. No further major medical or surgical interventions are planned, including resuscitation when the heart stops or placement of a breathing tube when breathing becomes insufficient. We stop all measures that maintain a very unstable medical situation and that could prolong the natural dying process. Doing everything possible is wrong when a person clearly is dying. We have to explain this to family members, even though it's a very delicate topic.

When aggressive care stops, palliative care begins, defined by physicians Claire Creutzfeldt, Benzi Kluger, and Robert Holloway in their book, *Neuropalliative Care,* as follows: "Palliative care is specialized medical care that aims to recognize, prevent, and alleviate physical, social, psychological, and spiritual suffering and improve communication about end of life and quality of life for patients with serious illness and their families."

Today, many palliative care specialists have extended their involvement beyond the last few days of life to the last few months of life. Their goal is to provide an environment of optimal comfort, acceptable symptom management, sufficient energy and peace of mind.

Palliative care is a developing medical specialty and far more complex than you might realize. Palliative care involves identifying and resolving distressing symptoms as well as supporting family members as they cope with a difficult situation. The overarching goal is to relieve suffering for both the dying individual and family members.

Neuropalliative care is similar but also recognizes differences of care among individuals with neurologic disease. In people with cancer, for example, treatment of symptoms is at the core of palliative care. In neurology, comatose individuals don't experience pain, hunger or thirst. Our palliative treatments are mainly focused on addressing insufficient breathing and general care once the person is no longer intubated.

In addition, much of the work of neuro-palliative care specialists involves helping families understand the process of dying. Even if an individual is deeply unconscious, it's very difficult for families (and for us as well) to observe physical responses and reflexes that can accompany dying, including grimacing, gasping, twitching in the face and body, tears, extended coughing spells, and moaning. The health care team will address these responses if they persist or worsen.

Physicians mention palliative care cautiously because of its clear historical connotation with the ending of life. As I discuss in previous chapters, withdrawal of care only occurs in a minority of patients admitted to intensive care units (ICUs), and only an estimated 1 in 10 patients with a severe, catastrophic brain injury loses all function. Withdrawal of care is more common in individuals who are persistently comatose after severe traumatic brain injury or severe stroke. Many factors other than the patient's medical situation play a role in determining when to initiate palliative care.

In this chapter, I go over the process of withdrawal, including medications used to address comfort and when and why we give them. It's important that family members receive information about this process and how their loved one's comfort will be maintained.

INITIATING THE END-OF-LIFE DISCUSSION

Unfortunately, family members sometimes need to make very difficult decisions after hearing about a loved one's prognosis. These decisions often come after learning what the future likely will hold for a loved one. Few people want to be confined to a bed, fed by tubes, have their urine drained with a catheter, and constantly be at risk of open pressure wounds. When we come to the conclusion that, realistically, that's the way a patient will live out life, we discuss this with family members and give them time to consider the situation.

Some families refuse to let nature take its course and choose to maintain current care. Postponing or completely avoiding a decision to discontinue aggressive care is often linked to strong personal and cultural beliefs. This type of response is also more likely if the coma is the result of a criminal assault or when there's anger within the family or anger directed at the health care team.

This decision may be a bit easier if a loved one is quite old, and it's definitely very difficult if the individual is relatively young. Care rarely is withdrawn in the case of comatose children and young adults simply because their brains have tremendous recuperative capacity and physicians can't predict exactly how these individuals will do.

There are certain situations, however, in which it's clear that recovery is out of the question. These situations include multiple failed treatments for brain cancer, massive hemorrhage in the brain, severe trauma with injury to many parts of the brain, and severe brain injury as a result of oxygen and blood pressure deprivation, such as after a suicide attempt.

Ending treatment vs. active euthanasia

It's important to clarify that stopping life-sustaining treatment is not the same as active euthanasia. The American Academy of Neurology (AAN) emphasizes a patient's right to refuse life-sustaining treatment. Neurologists are obligated to honor requests to withdraw or withhold care and to provide palliative care. The

AAN supports discontinuation of treatments that provide no benefit to a patient, including nutrition and hydration.

But it's not a neurologist's duty to provide assisted suicide or active euthanasia at the request of a patient or the patient's proxy. In the United States and most other countries, when anyone (competent or incompetent) requests euthanasia, a neurologist must insistently refuse.

Moreover, the line between active euthanasia (physician intent to cause death) and aggressive use of medications to provide comfort (physician intent to relieve perceived suffering) mustn't be blurred by prescribing extremely high doses of opioids. If there's no medical justification, high doses easily can be misconstrued as a concealed attempt to induce death. I revisit this later.

The emergence of euthanasia poses a major threat to the delicate process through which we labor to decide what's right and good and how comfort care is practiced throughout the world. Our desire to do good, along with shared decision-making, sometimes creates an unworkable environment for physicians who treat patients with certain catastrophic neurologic conditions. End-of-life care in the United States has become politicized and shaded with opinions of all kinds; it provides fodder for platitudes and can create a no-win situation for everybody involved.

In the United States, end-of-life care has been associated with so-called death panels, reflecting a mistaken concern about a hypothetical adjudicating body (panel) that apportions treatment and thus determines who gets another chance at improvement and who does not.

Is hastening death the same as causing death, irrespective of the method employed or the timeline during which it occurs? Some people equate voluntary withholding of food and fluids with physician-assisted suicide. Their reasoning is representative of a conservative religious viewpoint expressed in a set of Jewish, Christian and Islamic beliefs that prevail in much of the world outside of Western Europe and North America. It would be a mistake to put the differing moral perspectives that emerge from these religious traditions into one ethical framework.

In 2017, after years of legal and professional warring, the American College of Physicians (ACP) concluded that, "On the basis of substantive ethics, clinical practice, policy, and other concerns articulated in this position paper, the ACP doesn't support legalization of physician-assisted suicide. It is problematic given the nature of the patient-physician relationship, affects trust in the relationship and in the profession, and fundamentally alters the medical profession's role in society." It added "just as medicine cannot eliminate death, medicine cannot relieve all human suffering."

Strong, unwavering proponents of physician-assisted suicide may believe that the degree of suffering on the part of patients and their loss of dignity is underestimated. Polls suggest that a growing proportion of the population supports physician-assisted suicide (mostly outside a hospital setting) and even active euthanasia (mostly in a hospital setting), if given a choice. Physician-assisted death is currently available to the 1 in 6 Americans living in states where it's legal. In most cases, patients are prescribed lethal medications to be ingested at home. In states where assisted death in the hospital setting is allowed, most physicians don't participate.

In opinion surveys, Americans are very divided. One-third feel these decisions are within a patient's and family's purview, one-third oppose it under any circumstances, and the remaining one-third think it should be reserved for isolated cases. The main consequence of these divisions, which have remained constant over many decades, is that extreme positions are unlikely to become the norm and euthanasia will not generally be at the discretion of the individual.

Legal challenges to decisions involving physician-assisted suicide will continue, and some states, such as Oregon, are more accommodating than others. The issue likely will remain contentious. Efforts to educate more older adults about living wills may take precedence. Updating these documents to provide more information specific to health care is another priority. In this day and age, it's disheartening that we've not made further progress in the use and interpretation of advance directives.

Studies indicate that minority groups are less likely than whites to engage in any

type of end-of-life planning and less likely to have an advance directive or a health care proxy. Studies have also found that deeply religious individuals are less likely to engage in end-of-life planning, possibly because they feel that only God has the authority to determine the end of life. Some people also believe that having an advance care directive on file at the hospital might mean they'll receive poorer quality medical care. These are issues that we currently confront and will likely continue to confront in the future.

Now that I've explained what palliative care isn't — it's not active euthanasia or physician-assisted suicide — I want to make a case for good palliation and explain its aspect of care. We don't hasten a patient's departure, but we do ease any pain and discomfort.

THE FINAL DAYS

Withholding critical care means avoiding resuscitative measures, including dialysis, tracheostomy or gastrostomy, as well as withholding insulin infusion and certain medications including antibiotics and drugs that raise blood pressure (vasopressors or inotropes). Once the decision is made to withhold care or provide only palliative measures, there are potentially four pathways to death: in the ICU, on a non-ICU floor, in a hospice facility or at home. Many hospitals and in-house palliative care programs don't have separate hospice hospital or ward beds.

The chart on page 110 lists which procedures are generally discontinued and which the patient will continue to receive.

Often, the decision is made not to intervene when a complication occurs. For example, if a patient's blood pressure drops, we may treat it initially but won't escalate care by giving more medication. If a life-threatening infection occurs, we don't give antibiotics. If the kidneys stop working, we don't start dialysis. If the heart develops severe rhythm disturbances, we don't aggressively treat it with pacemakers or attempt to shock it into a normal rhythm. We don't initiate tracheostomy or gastrostomy procedures.

Finally, we don't resuscitate or place a patient on a ventilator if the heart stops.

These decisions should be driven purely by an individual's current state of illness and not necessarily based on age or previous medical conditions. However, nothing is etched in stone, and if someone improves unexpectedly and a better outcome may be possible, measures aimed at de-escalating care can be reversed.

When the decision is made to withhold critical care, it's very important to discuss with family members if this should be done gradually or more quickly.

Intensive Care Unit	Escalating Life-Sustaining Support	De-escalating Life-Sustaining Support	Withdrawal of Life-Sustaining Support
Brain catheter	+	+	−
Cardiopulmonary resuscitation	+	−	−
Mechanical ventilation	+	+/−	−
Antibiotics	+	−	−
Dialysis	+	+/−	−
Tracheostomy/ percutaneous gastrostomy	+	+	−
Readmission intensive care unit	+	−	−

This chart shows what type of care is withdrawn or can be withdrawn when life-sustaining therapy proves ineffective. The + sign means the measure, treatment or procedure continues, and the − sign means it's withdrawn. A +/- sign means it may or may not continue.

Abrupt measures include removing the ventilator and removing any other support system, such as a temporary pacemaker. "Pulling the plug" is truly an awful phrase and does not describe what we do. When a patient is removed from a ventilator and medication infusion is stopped, death will occur quickly and peacefully — but only if other organ systems have failed.

About half of the sickest individuals in a neurologic ICU will die within hours after support is withdrawn. Some may continue to breathe calmly and quietly and remain relatively stable awhile longer until the heart stops. Withdrawal of care can also be done in increments. This allows events to take their course without counteractive intervention.

Once we withdraw an individual from a respirator and are confident the individual will remain comfortable, the patient is generally transferred to a non-ICU room. Shortly after the respirator stops, the individual's breathing may speed up before it slows and becomes shallow. Snoring and rattling breathing can be alleviated by certain devices and medication, or by repositioning the body. Changed breathing sounds or development of a rattle usually indicate that death will occur within 24 hours.

Once an individual's breathing stops, color drains and the skin takes on a grayish-blue tone. The heart also soon stops beating, although it may take about five minutes to do so completely. The heart may even restart after a minute but with no measurable blood pressure.

Involving hospice

If death doesn't occur relatively quickly and it appears the individual may hold on for days, he or she may be transferred to a hospice facility. Many people survive for several days, which can be very hard on their families. Hospice is a special place with highly experienced staff, where a loved one and family members are made comfortable and supported. Some hospices are better than others. To my knowledge, good hospice experiences far outweigh negative ones. Hospice staff deserve the highest praise for providing care under often difficult circumstances.

We have no good way to predict how long it may take a comatose individual to find eternal rest, but we don't expect it to be more than 10 days. Although very little has been published about comatose patients dying at home, they require a certain level of nursing support to maintain hygiene and avoid overburdening family members with care that most family members aren't equipped to provide. A patient's physical, emotional, spiritual and psychological needs are often best met by a hospice team.

While caring for a loved one at home with family at the bedside may seem ideal, there are many details involved, and getting them all right can prove difficult. The chart on pages 112-113 summarizes key parts of reviews done by palliative care providers when they're called in to care for a patient. The chart is detailed and lengthy. Its purpose here is to emphasize the complexity of palliation.

Assessment of capacity for complex decision-making

- The first question will be if your loved one has the capacity to make complex medical decisions in the current setting. When the answer is no, the default is to the substituted decision-making process.
- Based on conversations with loved ones, the medical provider will make a judgment about who appears to be acting in a patient's best interests and keeping with the patient's known preferences.

Goals of care

- Code status: Do not resuscitate/do not intubate (DNR/DNI)
- Continuation of symptom-only management to allow for natural death
- Discontinuation of all life-prolonging therapies
- No escalation of care to the ICU (no blood pressure drugs, no breathing machines)
- No further rehospitalization
- No further labs, imaging or workups
- No antibiotics
- No artificial nutrition (no tubes)
- No dialysis
- Plan to enroll in hospice services upon discharge

Hospice discussion

Goals of care continue to align with the hospice philosophy:

- Eligibility generally is determined by a progressive decline in a patient in the context of overall health with a life expectancy of less than six months if the disease takes its natural course.
- Eligibility for general inpatient hospice is largely determined by the need for frequent medication adjustments, which may change if a patient's symptoms become difficult to control after withdrawal of care.

Legal and regulatory aspects of care/advance care planning documents

- Advance directive, including a detailed assessment of patient wishes on file, which can be used by staff to reach consensus
- Understanding of the meaning of terminal, which doesn't necessarily mean that death from the disorder is imminent

Pharmaceutical comfort care management

For pain or other signs of discomfort:
- Oxycodone
- Hydromorphone
- Morphine, starting at a low dose

Severe shortness of breath

- Initiation of oxygen therapy
- Diuretics such as furosemide to aid in labored breathing associated with fluid in the lungs

Fluids

- Provide education regarding artificial fluids at end of life. Complications of too much fluid may include edema, abdominal swelling, nausea, increased secretions and prolonging the dying process.
- Initiate nonpharmacological treatments, including use of bedside fan.
- For dry mouth, use of lip balm, mouth swabs or sips of water as tolerated.

Urinary retention

- Bladder scan.
- If retention develops, recommend urinary catheter at the end of life.

Constipation

- Polyethylene glycol 3350
- Medications containing bisacodyl if no bowel movement for more than two days
- Hold bowel regimen for frequent or loose stools (more than three a day)
- Education on the importance of continuing bowel regimen for opioid-induced constipation

Nausea and vomiting

- Continued monitoring
- Ondansetron

Agitation and delirium

- Nonpharmacological interventions.
- Rule out urinary retention and constipation.
- Maintain sleep-wake cycle by keeping blinds open, lights on and patient awake during the day as much as possible. Cluster care to promote rest and sleep at night.
- Frequent verbal redirection and orientation to surroundings, date and time (whiteboard and clock).
- Limit stimuli that may contribute to worsening symptoms, such as excess noise and conversation.
- Avoid physical tethers, such as any restraints, lines or monitors that aren't medically necessary.
- If nonpharmacological interventions aren't effective or if patient is harmful to self or others, recommend pharmacological treatment.
- Antipsychotic drugs such as haloperidol or risperidone.

Fever management

- Recommend cooling measures, such as a fan, ice packs, cooling blanket or cool, wet washcloth over skin.
- Acetaminophen.

Secretions

- Encourage upright positioning as much as tolerated (minimum 30-degree angle) to assist with clearing of secretions.
- Eliminate IV fluids to assist with fluid balance.
- No deep suctioning, given potential to promote gag reflex or vomiting.
- Atropine 1% ophthalmic solution.
- Glycopyrrolate.

THE DYING PROCESS

Dying is not a struggle in individuals who are unconscious; I can't overemphasize this. Any suggestion to the contrary is irrational. After everything is removed, these individuals pass quietly in a matter of days, and sometimes the same day that all life-support devices are withdrawn.

We don't provide fluids or food because we know they don't feel thirst or hunger. Family members often ask me about that, and I tell them that when a patient is deeply comatose or only minimally conscious, normal sensations simply disappear. (If you've ever had a bad case of the flu, you may remember not wanting to drink or eat.) Withdrawal of food and fluids results in death from dehydration, but there's no evidence that comatose patients sense thirst. In fact, fluids may cause them discomfort due to increased body water and gastric and pulmonary secretions. (See the Frequently Asked Questions section later in this book.)

The person's eyes eventually will close, and sleep-wake cycles will stop. Within days, urine production will slow or stop. This can cause increased acidity, which leads to increased breathing, the body's natural way of compensating. Even if breathing sounds more labored, the individual isn't actually in distress. Sometimes doctors may prescribe additional morphine if breathing becomes labored or there's rattling with a lot of secretions. Generally, though, it's not necessary. Withdrawal of care usually is sufficient in bringing about death.

A dying person's hands and feet will become cold to the touch due to poor circulation. The person's pulse will become weaker and barely palpable. Drying of mucous membranes can be minimized with mouth swabs and eye-drops. Facial features may change due to fluid loss, and the person may become more unrecognizable, which can be distressing to family members.

Over the years, I've heard and read concerns that individuals who are dying of dehydration have bleeding gums, parched lips, burning of the bladder from concentrated urine and difficulty breathing due to pooling mucus. I've never seen that in my patients, nor have the many other health care professionals with whom I've discussed it. I assure families that death is dignified and humane.

Comatose patients aren't wild or delirious after withdrawal of care. Many families remain at the bedside, and for most of them, having made the decision to withdraw care is a relief. In my experience, very few families have second thoughts about this step. Obviously, that outcome can only occur if they feel well informed and they trust the health care staff caring for their loved one.

Medications used

When caring for individuals in whom treatment is being withdrawn, experienced palliative care nurses should have wide latitude to give soothing medication as needed. The double effect of sedation is a major topic of discussion among bioethicists. The concern is that a potent sedative (or anesthetic) drug given to relieve distress may also hasten death because of an individual's inability to adequately breathe or maintain an airway while heavily sedated.

Some speak of "good" and "bad" effects. A good effect would be "morally good" — our guts say it's the right thing to do. A bad effect would be expected and unavoidable — "it is what it is" — when there are no better options. Administration of a sedative drug must meet the challenge of having the good outweigh the bad. For example, the ease in discomfort that's provided outweighs that fact that it may theoretically hasten death. A good effect, however, cannot come from a bad action.

I narrow the use of palliative medications depending on a patient's condition (see the table below). Medications are administered freely, if needed, to individuals who are drowsy, and they aren't given if brain death has occurred. An overdose of morphine will stop breathing and hasten death, but in terminal care, the dosage is carefully monitored and increased over time. Used in this way, the drug doesn't slow or stop breathing. In fact, in dying patients, small amounts of morphine are effective for treating distress associated with breathlessness.

We use minimum doses of morphine and anti-anxiety medications (benzodiazepines) as necessary to achieve patient comfort. Often, we start a morphine infusion to resolve grimacing or labored breathing and gradually increase the dosage. A benzodiazepine drug can be increased slowly until symptoms of agitation or restlessness are controlled. In deeply comatose individuals, this might not be

USE OF PALLIATIVE MEDICATIONS IN SPECIFIC NEUROLOGICAL STATES

	Drowsiness	Coma	Brain Death
Strong pain medications, such as opioids	+	−	−
Calming medication, such as benzodiazepines	+	−	−
Medication to prevent seizures	+/−	+/−	−
Medication to prevent secretions and nausea and vomiting	+	+	−

+ used; − avoided; +/− may or may not be used

necessary unless breathing after extubation becomes markedly labored.

In our institution, it's common practice to start a morphine infusion and increase the dosage in small increments every 15 minutes until a patient is free of pain. We may also do the same thing with the sedative drug lorazepam, adjusting it until we're able to control an individual's agitation or restlessness. None of this is indicated for deeply comatose patients unless their breathing becomes markedly labored after being removed from a respirator.

We always let families know that the starting doses may not be enough to prevent suffering, particularly in a person who has partially recovered from a coma. None of these drugs instantly alleviates distress. Relief sometimes doesn't occur until analgesics and sedatives reach their peak effects.

Treating respiratory distress

The clinical signs of respiratory distress are restlessness, moaning, agitation and changes in vital signs. Even when they're present, however, we can't be sure that a person is suffering. Conversely, even when patients are unable to express discomfort, they may still be aware of it.

This is why we have a strategy for providing compassionate care in patients no longer on a respirator who've recovered some awareness. Medications are adjusted until the person seems comfortable and there

are no apparent signs of suffocation, breathlessness or anxiety.

The sedative medication midazolam is the drug of choice for compassionate extubation. Another medication that may be used is the anesthetic propofol. Much has been written about the adverse effects of propofol, including deep sedation and impairment of breathing, but those concerns are misplaced when an individual is likely to die within a couple of hours.

Many ICUs prohibit the use of propofol in patients who aren't intubated, and the dosages recommended for those who are intubated are too low to be effective. Therefore, experienced palliative care physicians will likely start with midazolam and add fentanyl to ease any pain. This drug combination results in quiet sedation.

Treating other symptoms

After a patient's breathing (endotracheal) tube is removed, the person may or may not breathe. The deepest emotional responses of family members tend to occur when the tube is removed, making way for acceptance. We position the patient to facilitate airflow, and care providers may frequently need to suction mucus from the airway. Administering supplemental oxygen isn't beneficial and doesn't relieve symptoms.

Breathing may be noisy and rattling (agonal), and it may cause great distress to family members. (The word *agonal* often is misinterpreted as agony, but the actual definition is "relating to the act of dying.") If repositioning the person's head and body doesn't alter the breathing, we may administer the medications glycopyrrolate or scopolamine. Glycopyrrolate reduces saliva and drooling. Scopolamine relaxes the smooth muscles, and both drugs dry up secretions from the exocrine glands. Dry mouth is managed with oral hygiene every 2 to 4 hours, smoothing the lips with petroleum jelly, and moistening the air.

A number of other steps are taken in advance to prepare for things that can happen to the body when a patient is dying. Vomiting from increased intracranial pressure may be treated with medications to control vomiting (antiemetics). Hiccups can be relieved with the medication baclofen.

Extreme agitation can be treated with the medication lorazepam or the medications midazolam or propofol. Medications may also be administered to prevent seizures. Irregular shaking in all muscle groups (vigorous myoclonus) is very distressing to watch, and several anesthetic drugs administered in low doses can treat this.

It's important to discuss all of these end-of-life comfort measures with family members. I tell them the names of the medications and what they do, even if the names sound daunting. Otherwise, family members may misunderstand what we're trying to do or wonder if our actions are in their loved one's best interests. We go so far as to obtain consent from family members for use of the drugs so there are no misunderstandings.

Other considerations

There are other important considerations when care is withdrawn. All unnecessary equipment in their rooms should be disconnected and displays removed, although monitoring continues remotely. Noise and light in their rooms should be minimized. Chairs and tissues should be available for family members.

Physicians may be present, but they're often silent and respectful. Historically, in our institution, the only visible indicator that the individual was dying was a closed curtain. After death, a "Do not enter" (stop) sign was hung up or a staff member let colleagues know before they entered. My colleagues and I thought that was insufficient, and we introduced pictures of candles (see page 118).

When people see the pictures, they often pause, become silent and reflect. Candles have immense religious symbolism, but they also evoke peace, quiet and tranquility in the absence of any faith or belief system. They're neutral, universal symbols. We've found that posting these signs significantly reduces the noise level, particularly from staff conversations. The candle photos have been so well received that they're now being used in all ICUs in our hospital.

We don't pretend that these pictures alleviate the bereavement process, but the response to this simple gesture has been overwhelmingly positive. These placards are only used when individuals have transitioned to comfort care, their families have come to full agreement about withdrawal of support, and doctors anticipate a brief dying process.

We provide other measures, such as dimming of lights to create a calm atmosphere. We encourage families to bring to the bedside favorite items, such as photos, religious articles or quilts. We allow soft music and may prop a patient's head up with a favorite pillow or wrap the patient in a favorite blanket or quilt, if there is one. There also may be agreed-upon spiritual ceremonies.

Many hospitals, and their ICUs in particular, also have reflection rooms. These rooms offer a quiet place for family members to

sit, gather their thoughts, reflect, and let go of their emotions. Reflection rooms are usually peaceful and quiet, similar to a chapel. Reflection rooms can also be a place where chaplains visit with family members.

In many U.S. hospitals, a representative from the Office of Decedent Affairs (ODA) meets with family members of patients who have died. If there's a possibility that a death was not due to natural causes, the individual's personal belongings are considered evidence and placed in paper bags. The belongings can only be released to family members with authorization from the police and medical examiner. In these cases, the ODA representative will obtain written permission from the patient's legal next of kin for a postmortem examination. If next of kin aren't present and the patient had no

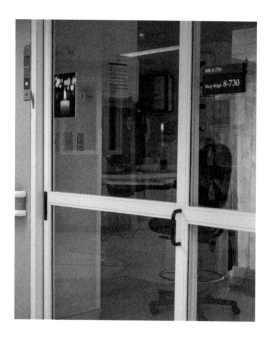

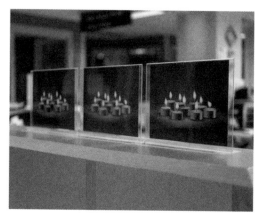

Photos of candles on a door to a patient room and at the nurse's station serve as simple and discreet visual reminders that a patient has shifted from life-sustaining interventions to end-of-life care.

advance directive, permission will be obtained through a recorded phone call.

An autopsy then will be performed within three months. The hospital is required to send an autopsy report to family members. The cause of death and what led to it are rarely a surprise, but the information may provide an opportunity for family members to discuss with physicians any uncertainties about what the final, definitive diagnosis means.

BEREAVEMENT

In her book *On Death and Dying*, Dr. Elisabeth Kübler-Ross concluded that there are five stages at the end of life: denial, anger, bargaining, depression and acceptance. Some people go through these stages, but for many others, grief may endure until a veil lifts. When that will happen can't be predicted.

The term *complicated grief* is used when yearning for a loved one is persistent and the person grieving withdraws socially and is preoccupied by the loss. Although fewer than 1 in 10 people experiences this type of grief, it can wreck a person's life if the symptoms aren't managed. Parents grieving the death of a young adult are at increased risk of physical and mental deterioration including depression that may necessitate hospitalization.

It's crucial that health care staff retain their humanity, treat patients and family members as individuals, and make decisions that respect their values. Bereavement-associated post-traumatic stress disorder (PTSD) occurs more frequently in families of individuals who die in the ICU. Studies performed in neurointensive care units show that 30% of family members who participate in end-of-life decision-making have some form of PTSD that persists for up to six months.

Some family members reach a default position of skepticism and profound sadness. Sudden, unexpected waves of emotion with yearning, regret and ambivalence are not unusual. Family members may need grief counseling. We discuss that with them in detail early on, and then social workers follow up. Risk factors for prolonged grief include concurrent stressors and lack of social support. Families should know that support doesn't stop when they leave the hospital and that medical staff is available for a phone call or visit.

AND FINALLY

To recap, when it's clear that an individual who is comatose has reached the very final stages and that continuing the current level of care would cause medically unjustifiable harm, family members and health care providers often stop aggressive treatment and turn to comfort (palliative) care. Once that decision is made, the health care team often will discuss with the family members whether life-sustaining care is withdrawn gradually or suddenly. During palliative care, the goal of medical professionals is to make patients as comfortable as possible and to prepare families for what they can expect as the dying process unfolds.

7

When is organ donation considered?

A CONVERSATION

Physician: Unfortunately, there's nothing more we can do for your son. His blood pressure was very low overnight and he's not moving. We think his brain is no longer functioning, and without support, he wouldn't breathe or have a blood pressure. We need to do a careful examination to find out where we are, but it's possible that he has already passed on.

Family: You've expressed your concerns and warned us this was very possible. Can we donate his organs? His driver's license indicates that he wanted to donate.

Physician: That's something we'll consider. You can meet with an organ donation representative after we've completed our examination. I'm so sorry for your loss, but rest assured, we tried everything. Maybe something good can come out of this tragedy and your son can save lives.

Family: That's what we'd like. Can we be there when you do your examination?

Physician: First let me explain what we'll do. Then you can decide if you want to be there.

Most individuals who suffer an acute catastrophic injury to the brain need to be placed on a ventilator. Many never improve. About 1 in 10 individuals treated in a specialized neuroscience intensive care unit (ICU) ultimately lose all brain function. We call this *brain death*, and it represents irrevocable loss of function in a person's brainstem. Allow me to provide some detail so you can better understand this condition.

BRAIN DEATH

As mentioned earlier, the brain has two halves (hemispheres), together called the cerebrum. The cerebellum and brainstem are located below the cerebrum. The brainstem connects the hemispheres with the spinal cord. Decades ago, scientists considered the brainstem nothing more than a "bridging" structure, but we now know that the brainstem controls all vital functions of the brain and is absolutely the most important structure in it. This understanding came about in the 20th century, and the significance of this radically different insight cannot be overstated.

Considering its enormous importance, it's astounding that the brainstem rarely is shown in diagrams of the brain in school textbooks or popular magazines. The brainstem awakens us and keeps us awake, and it also regulates everything else that supports life including the ability to recognize yourself and your surroundings. It holds the keys to breathing, maintaining a blood pressure, having muscle function, swallowing, moving your eyes, grimacing and making other facial movements, and registering touch and pain.

In short, brain death is massive damage to the brain's hemispheres followed by terminal brainstem injury. Once the brainstem stops functioning, recovery is

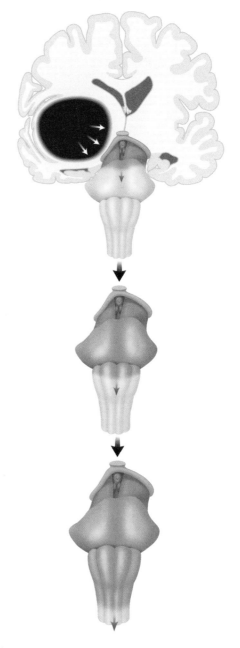

This illustration shows a mass that is compressing on and displacing the brain. The brainstem gradually loses its function in a vertical direction, as indicated.

impossible, and a person has passed the point of no return. Often, brainstem function is lost gradually, from the top down, until there's nothing left (see the illustration).

To repeat what I said in Chapter 1, brain death differs from a vegetative state. In a vegetative state, the cerebrum is damaged, but the brainstem remains largely intact, allowing breathing and blood pressure to continue independently. A patient in a vegetative state may recover, although it's exceptionally rare. I can't emphasize enough that viability of the brainstem is key to our understanding of acute injuries to the brain. It's far too easy to confuse a vegetative state and brain death, even among health care staff. That's because on the surface, these conditions appear to be the same.

When comatose patients who become brain dead arrive at a hospital, they're often in very bad shape. Suddenly, all their movements, including primitive reflexes, may stop. Their muscle tension is gone, and they're floppy and flaccid. They no longer respond to suctioning of secretions, and their blood pressure drops. Keeping such patients at a level sufficient to maintain heart and kidney function requires medication. In brief, without aggressive life support, the body will decline quickly, and the heart will stop.

We have the ability to use machines to keep patients with almost any life-threatening medical condition alive. But this can't continue indefinitely. Eventually — often after weeks, if life support continues — a patient's heart will stop.

DEFINING DEATH

When physicians talk about death, we have to weigh our words carefully. Saying that "the patient died" is medically correct, but many people only accept death if there's no heartbeat, blood circulation or breathing.

A person dies when the brain or heart stops functioning. When the brain stops, the heart stops, and when the heart stops, the brain stops. We can try to jump-start the brain (breathing machine and blood pressure drugs) or heart (chest compression and drugs), but often it's too late for that. Once the brain, specifically the brainstem, is dead, we cannot revive it.

Determining that a person is brain dead requires an extensive evaluation, as described in Chapter 1. Most of the time, we test all reflexes and try to stimulate the individual's breathing centers.

Some experts believe it's valuable to have family members witness the examination, particularly if it helps them realize that their loved one has died. Gaining a better understanding of brain death and how it's diagnosed with simple tests may remove any doubts they have, and it provides transparency. Other experts contend that having family members present causes families too much distress.

In any case, I offer families the opportunity and explain the tests I'll be doing. They include applying hard pressure to the patient's face, arms and legs, squirting ice water in the ears, complete removal from the ventilator for 8 to 10 minutes, and several blood draws. In my experience, few family members want to watch all of that being done to a loved one. I'm also not sure that those who have watched me have found it helpful. I know for sure, however, that some of them didn't like what they were seeing, even though they understood that these tests were necessary.

A declaration of brain death is made methodically, carefully, slowly, and with great deliberation and consultation. Once an individual is declared brain dead, we'll discuss the implications with family members. At this point, there's no need to continue mechanical ventilation or to maintain blood pressure support. Families usually understand that removing this support makes complete sense. We may delay it if other family members need to arrive and say their goodbyes. It's probably easier to say goodbye while the support is still in place, rather than after a body has lost all form of life.

Families may decide not to be present when support is withdrawn or arrive after the process is complete. Removal of the ventilator is simple when it's readily apparent that the individual can't breathe. Oxygen levels fall and blood pressure disappears. The heart stops pumping, and its electrical activity stops after 5 to 10 minutes. Support isn't withdrawn, however, before families speak to an organ donation representative.

REFERRAL FOR ORGAN DONATION

If family members know that their loved one was interested in organ donation, we refer them to an organ-donation procurement officer. A patient's wish to be an organ donor may be expressed on a driver's license, or the individual may be listed in other donor registries. In the United States, you can register as an organ donor with Donate Life America.

The Uniform Anatomical Gift Act allows families in the United States to donate a loved one's entire body for transplantation or research. This can include organs and also the corneas in the eyes and other tissues, such as skin and bone. Rarely is a donor's full hand, face or uterus transplanted by surgeons. A surgeon must have extraordinarily specialized skills to perform such procedures. The consent for such donations is separate when a recipient is available. (As an aside, face transplantation doesn't make the recipient look like the donor, although there might be a slight, very superficial resemblance. The donated face adapts to the recipient's bone structure. The result differs significantly from both the original damaged face and the donor's face and, thus, often is referred to as the "third face.")

We have a legal obligation to put families in contact with an organ-donation agency so that a coordinator can explain what organ donation is and how it works. There are more than 50 organ-procurement organizations in the United States, and their coordinators are highly trained specialists who work with surgeons retrieving organs for transplantation.

Organ-procurement organizations are independent, private, nonprofit organizations. Each is assigned by the Health Care Financing Authority to a specific geographic area that comprises several states. All organ-procurement organizations are funded by the Health Care Financing Authority and by transplant centers that receive organs recovered by organ-procurement organizations. Organ-procurement organizations bill the receiving transplant center for the costs associated with organ transplantation. The donors' families pay nothing.

My opinion is that organ donation should only be discussed with a family after their loved one is brain dead or when the decision has been made to withdraw support and remove the ventilator from someone with an irrefutably irrecoverable brain injury. The point at which those two paths cross naturally leads to a conversation about possible organ donation with family members.

Because public education and experience with organ donation and transplantation have increased, more families are approaching physicians about donation options. This often happens before a patient is declared brain dead or has been removed from supporting medications and mechanical ventilation. Even if a family asks questions about donation, I believe it's better to postpone a detailed discussion and focus on explaining their loved one's current condition. But if a family really wants to have a conversation about organ donation, specific questions about the process should be answered.

Family members generally aren't connected with a transplant coordinator before a brain death examination has taken place. Delaying this in-depth discussion is somewhat controversial, and there may be a preference by organ-donation agencies to have everyone involved earlier. Many of my colleagues agree, however, that only when brain death is declared should a patient's family be considered ready for a discussion about donation and which organs and tissues can be donated.

I've found that too much information is overwhelming, and in the "limbo period" preceding a declaration of brain death, family members are often too confused to focus clearly. Therefore, I feel it's best to move slowly and deliberately.

ORGAN DONATION

Let me do my best to explain organ transplantation, a complex topic, as simply as possible. I'll start with a troubling statistic. Every day, an estimated 10 people in the United States die because organs aren't available to save their lives. Moreover, consent rates for donation by families are roughly 60% to 70%, which is reasonably high, but ideally, more organs are needed to prevent unfortunate deaths daily.

Organs aren't readily available for the taking. For eligible recipients, the waiting period to receive an organ is long, and often it's simply good luck when a recipient receives an organ in time. Organ donation and transplantation also involve an intricate infrastructure, close collaboration by several medical and surgical specialists, and collaboration with many health care providers. It's difficult for outsiders (and even many physicians in other medical specialties) to understand the enormity of the process, the logistics involved, the extreme efforts to maintain confidentiality, and the level of care taken.

Given all the waiting recipients, only rarely are donor organs and tissues found to be incompatible and no match possible, but incompatibility does limit the eligibility of some individuals. Some people mistakenly attribute an inability to achieve a match to bias or prejudice. That can lead to mistrust of and dissatisfaction with the organ donation system.

Not everyone supports organ transplantation. Some individuals and groups have given organ donation an unnecessarily bad reputation by portraying it as a $20-billion-per-year business and focusing on the high salaries of transplant surgeons. What's completely ignored is the tremendous complexity of the operations and the acts of great altruism and compassion from courageous family members of recently deceased loved ones. Criticizing or mocking these tremendous gifts is shocking.

Advances in transplantation

Saving a terminally ill patient by way of organ transplantation has been one of medicine's greatest success stories, a triumph that was considered unimaginable half a century ago. Success was achieved only after many stops and starts.

The early history of transplantation was marked by failure and frustration among pioneering surgeons and physicians, who tried repeatedly to improve the outcome with drugs that prevent the body from rejecting new organs (immunosuppressive medications).

The kidneys were the first organs used for transplantation attempts, followed by the liver and heart. Success with these procedures has increased over many decades. Recently, transplantations of the face, hands, shoulders, and arms have been performed. The latest advance is uterus transplantation, which has resulted in successful pregnancies for the recipients. Bowel and pancreas transplants also are relatively common and have become successful. It's hard to imagine what it means for transplant recipients to receive a second chance when an organ becomes available.

Today, organ transplantation can also be performed with live donors. Family members who are good matches for a recipient can donate a kidney or part of a liver, often with great success.

Making the donation decision

Public support for organ donation is very high, but many Americans don't register to be donors or check the box on their driver's license to indicate that they want to donate. In the absence of one of those actions, it's difficult for physicians and organ-procurement organizations to know an individual's preference, and the decision is relegated to family members, who may or may not know. Once family members have a reasonably good idea about what organ donation entails, they can decide whether to proceed.

In the United States, approximately 70% of close family members consent to donate the organs of eligible patients. The reasons family members object are many and varied. It may have to do with religious beliefs. Some feel uncomfortable with organ removal. Myths also may play a role. One myth is that organ removal makes an open-casket funeral impossible.

In many European and Latin American countries, organ transplantation is an opt-out system. Consent is assumed unless a patient's family files an objection, and that happens only 5% to 10% of the time. It took many of these countries at least 10 years to prepare for this bold move with public education and increased hospital capacity. There's no evidence, however, that the opt-out system has led to more transplants, even though it has increased the number of donors.

The benefits of organ donation are significant. As the saying goes, it's one of the greatest gifts a person can give, and organ donation recipients are immensely grateful. From what I've seen, families of organ donors are proud of supporting their loved ones' values and fulfilling their presumed wishes. I've never heard any of them express regrets; their experiences seem to be universally positive. Many of the families want to know how many organs were eventually transplanted, and the organ-donation agency often will inform them in a letter.

All of this said, a family's refusal to donate organs, after a detailed explanation of what's involved, should be accepted gracefully, and the family shouldn't be forced to explain their decision. Knowing donation can save lives may not be an overriding argument; some people simply want to bury their loved ones as they were upon death.

HOW THE PROCESS WORKS

Here are some important facts about organ transplantation it's helpful to know. The Health Care Financing Authority imposes several requirements on hospitals designed to increase organ donation. Hospitals must ensure, in collaboration with the organ-procurement organization with which they have an agreement, that the families of all potential donors are informed about the option to donate organs or tissues.

How should a conversation about organ transplantation take place and what, ideally, should a family expect to hear? First, it's important that the conversation not take place in a waiting room with the relatives of other patients. The family needs a calm place to reflect and grieve in privacy. Second, it's appropriate to explain that organ procurement is a long procedure, which can take 24 to 48 hours to complete. This has everything to do with finding a perfect match and ascertaining whether the donor's organs are, indeed, suitable.

Transplantation coordinators come to the hospital if the family wants to speak with them, but we're cautious about initiating conversations about transplantation if we think they might be premature.

In my experience, overwhelming family members with too much information about organ transplantation too early in the process — such as before a loved one is presumed brain dead — can leave family members confused, annoyed and even occasionally angry. Mending the relationship may require significant effort on the part of all stakeholders. My goal has always been to take it one step at a time and to avoid saying too much too soon.

Hospitals must agree to contact their assigned organ-procurement organization in a timely manner when a patient has died, or death is imminent. The call often is made when a do-not-resuscitate (DNR) order is in place, no surgical or other medical options are available, and recovery is absolutely ruled out. Individuals considered as organ donors often are close to being brain dead, and it's expected that testing will confirm brain death. In addition, hospitals must have an agreement with at least one tissue bank and one eye bank to cooperate in recovering, processing, preserving, storing, and distributing those organs, provided these measures don't interfere with organ donation.

The figure below and the shaded box on the right provide details on steps taken to verify donation eligibility. First, a full and comprehensive neurologic examination determines if the person is brain dead. Once that's complete, depending on the results, the ventilator can be removed, or organ donation can begin. If the person isn't brain dead, the family can continue care (short or long term), withdraw the

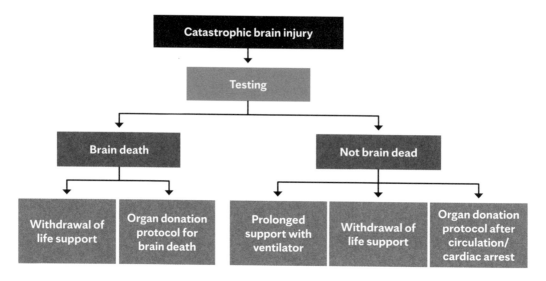

This algorithm outlines the process for determining eligibility for organ donation.

ventilator or start the process of organ donation. These options may seem complicated, and we take considerable time to explain them.

Several bedside tests and additional blood draws are necessary to determine which organ(s) can be used. It's not unusual that an individual's brain injury renders some organs unusable. The organ-procurement organization then determines, on a case-by-case basis, if the patient is medically suitable to be a donor and contacts the hospital when decisions have been made.

Once organs have been deemed suitable for donation and the surgical team is ready, the patient is transported to the operating room. Family members are informed of the time of transport well in advance and can be present to say their goodbyes until their loved one leaves for the operating room. Some people decide to say their goodbyes earlier because it can take up to two days before organ removal is performed.

Organ-procurement coordinators work closely with families to ensure that all the details and timing work for the family and for the surgeons. The organs are recovered by a trained transplant surgeon, but family members don't speak with that person. All conversations go through the trained organ-procurement representative.

Once the patient enters the operating room, a team of surgeons and surgical assistants proceed with surgery. As with any type of heart or belly surgery, it involves a large skin and bone incision. The organs are carefully preserved and packaged for the waiting recipient. The ventilator is then removed, and the deceased donor is transferred to the hospital morgue and, eventually, to a

DONATION PROCESS AFTER BRAIN DEATH

- Neurologist examines patient and pronounces brain death
- Neurologist speaks with the family and explains that the patient has passed on, but organ function is supported
- Organ transplant coordinator talks with family, explains the process of organ donation and obtains consent
- Organ transplantation coordinator takes over care and obtains studies to check suitability of organs (24-36 hours)
- Family members say their goodbyes
- When a match is found, the patient goes to the operating room for organ removal, where ventilator support is withdrawn
- Body sent to the morgue

funeral home, where the family can make funeral arrangements. This protocol is called donation after brain death (DBD).

As noted in the figure on page 128, there's another situation in which organ donation can be considered. An individual may not be brain dead but have a very severe injury from which there is no recovery. In these cases, a physician must be very certain that nothing more can be done and that the patient will never awaken. The family then can decide to remove all support and proceed with what we call comfort care measures, in which the ventilator is removed and medication given only if distress is apparent.

Anyone age 65 or younger is a potential candidate for organ donation in this circumstance. Withdrawal of life support is performed in the operating room, and the organs are removed when there's no measurable blood pressure.

Again, an organ-procurement coordinator meets with the family to answer questions and ask for consent. Upon consent, the search begins for a good match, which can take up to 36 hours. At the same time, bedside tests are performed, and blood and tissue samples may be taken from the comatose individual to ensure that the organs are suitable for transplantation.

DONATION PROCESS AFTER CARDIAC (CIRCULATORY) ARREST

- Neurologist examines patient and finds that the patient isn't brain dead but won't survive except with aggressive life support.
- Neurologist speaks with family and explains the patient won't recover. Family decides not to continue support, knowing recovery won't occur. If the patient is younger than age 65, organs can be donated.
- Organ-procurement coordinator talks with family, explains the process of organ donation and obtains consent.
- Organ-procurement coordinator takes over care and obtains studies to check suitability of organs (24-36 hours).
- Family can stay with the patient or leave earlier if they prefer.
- When a match is found, the patient (and family, if they wish) go to the operating room, where the ventilator is removed.
- The physician and family wait for up to an hour for breathing to stop and blood pressure to become unmeasurable (absent circulation). Patient is then declared dead, and the family leaves.
- A five-minute waiting period is instituted. Then the surgeons arrive and obtain the organs to be donated.
- Body sent to the morgue.

Donation after cardiac death

The process of donation after cardiac (circulatory) arrest is different. It's called the donation after cardiac death (DCD) protocol. The patient is fully draped in sterile blankets in the operating room, and instruments are prepared and placed on a tray. Family members can enter, if they want to, but the procedure is very difficult to witness. Family members are invited to sit close to the patient's head, behind a sterile drape, and then the ventilator is removed.

Everything is done to provide comfort to the patient, but the patient may gasp for several minutes before breathing stops. It also may take several minutes for blood circulation to stop. Once that occurs, the individual is declared dead by a separate physician in the room, and the family leaves the operating room.

After about five minutes of waiting, the surgical transplant team enters the room and opens the chest and belly to remove organs for transplantation. Just as families rarely watch an actual surgical procedure, the family can't be present during this procedure.

In approximately 1 in 3 patients, breathing continues when the ventilator is removed, and the circulation doesn't stop within an hour after removal. It's very hard to predict when this will occur. There are models that tell us when it's likely, but none are perfect. Families are forewarned that their loved one may return to the intensive care unit if this happens. Obviously, organs aren't removed from a still-breathing person with intact blood pressure.

Like donation after brain death, donation after cardiac death is a well-organized, coordinated procedure that takes time. The protocol increases the time in the hospital by a couple of days, which most families find an acceptable price, knowing the donation of organs can potentially help up to eight individuals on transplant lists. Many families also appreciate the extra hours with their loved one as a time to say goodbye.

In my many experiences with comatose patients, discussions regarding brain death don't come up very often, and I hope it's something your family won't have to experience. If your family must make a decision regarding organ donation, remember that it's an opportunity for something good to result from a tragedy.

What surveys have found

When families of donor patients are contacted later about the donation process, surveys suggest the responses are mostly positive.

One survey of about 100 families who donated at Hartford Transplant Center in Connecticut revealed that nearly all of them found the experience was satisfactory. Many indicated the main reason for their decision was to help others. Some indicated the donation added something positive to their tragedy and felt that the recipient would live a better life. A few wanted the donor to "live on" in someone else and considered the donation a memorial to their deceased loved one.

The survey also found that 1 in 3 families indicated their loved ones had previously expressed a desire to donate, which made their decisions easier. Of course, the results reflect only the opinions of the people who responded to the survey, but they confirm that most families find organ donation to be a good experience.

A broader review of the literature on the experience of organ donation reveals some recurring themes. At the time they're asked to donate, families are

10 FACTS YOU'LL HEAR DURING A CONVERSATION WITH AN ORGAN-PROCUREMENT COORDINATOR

1. We try everything, and organ donation is never on physicians' minds until the situation is truly hopeless and nothing more can be done.
2. Physicians and organ-donation agencies have completely different paths and meet only at the very end. This is both a legal and ethical issue that's carefully monitored by hospitals.
3. Organ donation is a very complex, time-consuming procedure. A national computer system matches the donor and recipient information, based upon blood type, time spent waiting on the list, age, size of organs and preexisting medical conditions, and not on social status or financial background.
4. Families can stay with a loved one until the patient goes to the operating room.
5. Organ donation can save up to eight lives and benefit up to 75 other individuals through tissue donation.
6. Cornea donation restores sight in more than 95% of all transplants and to more than 84,000 people each year.
7. Funeral arrangements won't be affected. An open casket and a viewing are still possible if your loved one is a donor.
8. The transplant organization will provide a detailed letter about which organs were donated and how many people received the organs, but the organ recipients are kept anonymous.
9. Transplant organizations can contact the recipients to ask if they want to meet the family of the donor. Some recipients agree to meet with the donor's family, and others choose not to.
10. The organ-procurement organization is responsible for all hospital costs, from time of authorization to completion of procurement. Funeral home decisions and costs are the family's responsibility.

overwhelmed with emotions, have difficulty grasping what's being said to them and often don't understand what brain death means.

Many of these concerns may reflect procedural differences across health care systems. A common issue is that the declaration of brain death often is unexpected, and it's the health care team's responsibility to prepare families carefully for this possible outcome.

No study has documented regret after donation. The opposite, unfortunately, is true. Some families later feel guilty about not donating a loved one's organs. These perspectives are useful to health care staff and can help us better support families.

BARRIERS TO ORGAN DONATION

I support organ donation to the fullest extent, but I also recognize the barriers to it. Some ethicists, religious leaders and even physicians are conscientious objectors to organs that are donated from individuals declared dead.

The perspectives of religious organizations regarding organ donation are unclear. All major Christian denominations, Judaism, Islam, Buddhism, and Hinduism are supportive of helping others and emphasize the great opportunity to save another person's life.

Nonetheless, some denominations don't seem to approve of donation, often due to the personal opinions of their religious leaders. In addition, certain religious

tenets, such as the Japanese Shinto religion, which considers a dead body to be impure, dangerous and still quite powerful, make it difficult for families to proceed with organ donation. In a diverse, multicultural world, differences of opinion are to be expected.

AND FINALLY

I'd be remiss if I didn't acknowledge the possibility that major conflicts about organ transplantation sometimes arise between families and members of the health care staff. Almost always, our staff has cordial relationships with families. Sometimes, a complete breakdown occurs, and a family loses trust in the physicians taking care of their loved one.

What do we do to help a family that wants to continue care against all odds? If they won't accept brain death as death, there are two options. The first is to consider maintaining full support for a patient for a few days while trying to resolve the situation. In that case, the physician should ask for assistance from a hospital ethics committee to explain to the family that brain death is, in fact, the death of a person. Spiritual counsel may become involved as having a member of the clergy present can be very helpful. A second option is to directly involve a judge. It's an option that we absolutely try to avoid.

Above all, it's important to be sensitive and to try to help family members reach a sense of closure. Whether disputes can be avoided with more effective communication or using a mediator to help resolve issues between health care staff and families remains to be studied. Transferring the patient to another institution isn't a good resolution.

I think there are several reasons why issues arise when the topic of organ donation is discussed:

- Physicians may not have provided family members with the information they needed to make an informed decision.
- The request for organ donation may occur prematurely or unexpectedly.
- Religious and cultural beliefs may not be fully recognized by health care staff.
- The family may be praying for a miracle or convinced that a miracle will come.
- Family members may be distrustful, angry or experiencing other emotions that prevent them from acknowledging the medical reality of the situation.
- Family members may worry that they're "giving up" on a loved one or making the wrong decision.
- There may be reasons of which we're unaware, such as dissatisfaction with the care their loved one has received.

It's important to educate families about the donation process, acknowledge the strain they're under, and describe the satisfaction of others who've contributed a loved one's organs. This may help them reach a decision. Giving a family time after the diagnosis of brain death to consider information about organ donation allows them to organize their thoughts and arrive at the conclusion that's best for them.

Certainly, some people's views will never change. But if we can keep families that are unsure about organ donation from buying into fallacies and misconceptions, then we've accomplished something and helped them to make an informed decision. If the family grants approval, transplant recipients who benefit by being given a second chance at life will be indescribably grateful.

Finally, people often are not aware that all patients who die in the hospital or in hospice can potentially donate their bodies as an "anatomical gift." However, this decision needs to be made earlier and cannot happen after a tragic accident.

An individual must choose anatomical whole-body donation and register for it in writing while still of sound mind. A whole-body donation is an unmeasurable benefit to medical students, who will learn more about anatomy from such a gift than from any textbook or diagram.

You may not have expected an elaborate discussion of organ donation in a book on coma, and again, in the greater scheme of things, the issue doesn't come up very often. But for many decades, and frankly as long as transplantation has existed, there's been a growing need for donated organs and tissue.

When it's clear that a dying person would have wanted to be an organ donor — based on prior conversations with family or possessing a donor card — family members can make a great gift on their loved one's behalf. And for the recipients of donated organs, transplantation offers a new lease on life; hence, the metaphor, "gift of life."

HONORING THE
Gift of Life

IN THE MAYO CLINIC MISSION OF PROVIDING HOPE AND HEALING TO OUR PATIENTS, WE HONOR PEOPLE WHO GIVE OF THEMSELVES TO SERVE OTHERS THROUGH SELFLESS ACTS OF DONATION.

ORGAN, BLOOD, EYE AND TISSUE DONATIONS PROVIDE NEW LIFE TO THEIR RECIPIENTS. ANATOMICAL DONATIONS ADVANCE THE TRAINING OF HIGHLY SKILLED, COMPASSIONATE HEALTH CARE PROFESSIONALS.

WITH THE GENEROUS SPIRIT OF THESE DONORS, EVERY LIFE HAS A NEW BEGINNING.

A Gift of Life commemoration in St Marys Hospital, on the Mayo Clinic Campus in Rochester, Minn.

What are our moral obligations and duties?

8

A CONVERSATION

Physician: We've reached a point where we need to consider what we can and can't achieve for your mother.

Family: There are days when we think she's getting better and recognizes us and other days when she doesn't react at all. If she could talk, we think she'd say, "Please let me go" or "Just end it, please." Should we really stop all treatment? That seems like killing her. She may look bad to you, but she's fooled us in the past.

Physician: Let me explain some options, and then we can talk about what's morally acceptable and what we can do for your mother.

Ethical (moral) concerns always linger in the back of physicians' minds when caring for comatose patients. These questions can take center stage in difficult situations when treatment options have clearly run out and when anything we do must seem unacceptable. Family members often will ask us what they should do, saying "This can't go on," expressing feelings of hopelessness. This isn't surprising, given how stressful, complicated and uniquely disruptive it can be for family to care for a loved one who's comatose. It's common for some ethical dilemmas to arise.

Most humans have a desire and a need to do good, and they can recognize what's intuitively wrong. When this duty "to do good" involves making personal judgments about the value of life, we must work from an agreement in moral matters — what is right and what is wrong. Along with the irrevocable loss of someone they love, family members have an obligation to honor their loved one's wishes.

Making decisions based on "gut reactions" should be avoided because the choices often can be irrational. Achieving moral compromises during family conferences is an important goal when caring for a comatose patient. This often takes commitment and time. As physicians, we constantly must ask ourselves if we're doing good rather than harm and if we're working from a highly balanced assessment of the situation.

Grasping the significance of what I'm trying to convey may be a little easier if I outline what I consider to be the most acceptable ethical approach to caring for a comatose patient. I'll focus on the personal side and not just philosophical theory. I don't pretend to offer solutions or extraordinary advice, but I will examine issues that worry physicians when we make ethical decisions. Because the issues involved are becoming ever more complex, it's easy to drift from reality into abstraction when discussing them.

WHAT IS NEUROETHICS?

Medical ethics can be summarized as the recognition of and the determination to resolve moral problems associated with the care of a patient (in our case, a comatose patient). This burden, ultimately, involves everyone striving to do their best. Doctors need to be careful not to be lackadaisical or to take an extreme position if it's not warranted. Coma, and certainly one that's prolonged, immediately invites questions about the goals of care.

The topic of futility may arise, but it's hard to define and grasp, and some ways of defining it are questionable. Futility may mean continuation of care despite a hopeless situation, not "letting nature take its course." It may be viewed as treatment that won't accomplish a set goal, or when the burdens, suffering and costs of treatment far exceed any benefit. Attempts to define futility in percentages of treatment success — such as less than a 1% chance of recovery — offer a loose definition and may appear arbitrary to physicians and, certainly, to family members. A person's outcome is never a simple statistic.

Although the determination of futility is imprecise, pragmatic judgments are necessary in daily medical practice. Without them, the patient, physician and family remain at a standstill. Medicine would become a corporate discipline if medically unnecessary treatments were given without serious critical reflection. It's useful to view futility in terms of a patient's progress (or lack thereof). Futility is when we determine that there's no possible way to reverse an individual's downward course and achieve a good outcome. Once that's established, we can adapt and provide a different type of care, such as palliative care. The aim is comfort. Remember that care of a patient never stops until there's finality and eternal rest.

Any possible course of action in medicine can lead to ethical questions. Whenever we take a position, some people will agree with it, and others will not. No matter which side you're on, ethics can't be viewed in terms of "black or white," "good or evil," or "right or wrong." We always must balance morals and values and recognize each other's good intentions.

Religion and culture play a role in the practice of ethics; however, most major religions and cultures, along with most of society, strongly support relief of suffering. Relief is achieved through pharmacological means or by ending all useless interventions. Strongly conservative religious beliefs deserve respect, but they shouldn't become the dominant ethical stance. Older traditions may give way to newer traditions or beliefs.

Physicians caring for comatose individuals and family members often must consider what level of care to provide (see the shaded box below). Questions about the neuroethics of these decisions — ethical or philosophical arguments about how best to manage serious neurologic diseases — are common. The goal always is preservation of — and not violation of — human dignity.

While still healthy, many patients inform family members that they don't want to be a burden to others if they became ill or are injured. Memories of these conversations often influence family members' preferences regarding aggressiveness of care. Of course, we can't confirm what was said, and seldom can we ask the individual because few patients in intensive care are able to make such decisions.

Providing continuous care to a loved one with a devastating brain injury with no hope for recovery or ever awakening from a coma, may seem futile to some people, but not to others. This is often where differences between physicians and family members originate. However, we fully empathize with the anguish of

LEVELS OF CARE TO CONSIDER WHEN SETTING LIMITS

- Maximal therapeutic effort with no restrictions on any type of intervention.
- Maximal therapeutic effort but only for a specific period of time with reassessment of whether adjustment is needed.
- Continuing care but without initiating active or specific therapy (such as transfusions or antibiotics). Supportive medical care also replaces major new measures (ventilators, cardiac pacemakers, dialysis). No cardiopulmonary resuscitation.
- Attention given to comfort, including oxygen therapy for shortness of breath and analgesics for relief of pain. If the patient improves, reclassification may occur.
- All therapy stopped and nursing continues.

seeing a beloved, energetic, fun-loving person become suddenly and permanently incapacitated.

When it comes to issues regarding care, health care staff know they may be on the receiving end of criticism. Questions such as, "Why are you doing that? Why aren't you doing more? Why are you hurting my mother? Why isn't anybody taking care of her?" are common. We understand that families of comatose patients are emotionally stretched to the breaking point despite our best efforts to support them as we care for their loved ones.

In earlier chapters, we already delved into some major ethical issues. The underlying theme of this chapter is that ethics must dictate all medical care. Physicians want to provide maximal care, but as compassionate human beings, we can't disregard a patient's or family's wishes that we stand down and let nature take its course, particularly if the request is legitimate.

DEFINING QUALITY OF LIFE

Certainly, there's no easy way to describe well-being, and all of us probably have

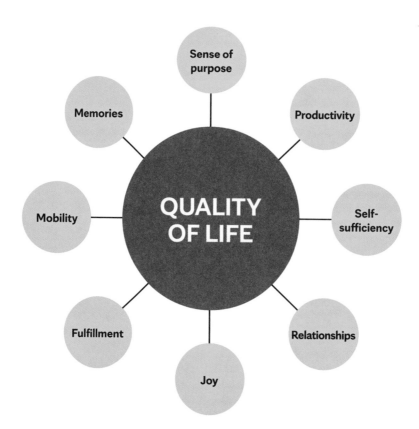

Factors that contribute to quality of life.

preconceived notions about what it involves. Ethics are tools to help interpret quality of life, a term that's not easy to define. There are just as many definitions of quality of life as there are people trying to define it.

Nevertheless, quality of life isn't completely incomprehensible, and most people wouldn't hesitate to label quality of life as being "low" for a person with no sense of purpose, who's dependent, is lonely, feels worthless, is immobile, can't recall recent events, and lives only in the moment (see illustration).

Yet no matter how good we think we are at describing quality of life, it's still a judgment call. It also may be quite relative and different for a person in a coma after a major brain injury than for someone born with a major brain dysfunction or with a slowly progressive neurologic disorder. Many comatose individuals had excellent (or at least, good) quality of life before the events that led to their comas.

The questions we ask about quality of life in a comatose individual are different. How much can he or she adjust? Can the person find meaning in life? Will the loss of many pleasurable and meaningful activities result in a joyless existence? I think we'd all agree that a life consigned to passive compliance, and in which one may be pitied and possibly ostracized, isn't dignified. We're fundamentally social creatures, and a major brain injury can change all that.

For physicians, quality of life often is measured in the absence of specific signs and symptoms, but we all know there's much more to be considered. Rehabilitation teams have created an abundance of quality-of-life scores. Some of these metrics work and others don't. Physicians should strongly reject scoring systems with cutoff values that determine whether a person makes the grade or not.

Family members, for example, may want to spare their loved one the indignity of full dependence on life-sustaining equipment. When they decide to withdraw care, they're not deliberately trying to induce death — anything but. They can do it because they know the individual well enough to understand what that person would have wanted, which should be the only motivation.

Physicians generally understand that we lack expertise regarding normality and abnormality when it pertains to quality of life. And we should avoid judging the meaning of life or deciding when life is miserable. We're very cautious about what we say in that regard, and rightly so.

When dealing with quality of life, we do better when we have less respect for rules and more respect for principles. For generations, a physician's words were accepted as final, correct and to be obeyed. However, we're not infallible. As health care staff, we acknowledge that we usually know very little about the lives of the patients we treat. To conclude that a person's quality of life is going to be unacceptable must be a consensus opinion in which no single person, including a physician, takes a dominant stance.

GUIDING PRINCIPLES

The core principles of neuroethics are closely linked to the basics of bioethics. Traditionally, the fundamentals of medical ethics have focused on four pillars advanced by Beauchamp and Childress: autonomy, justice, beneficence and non-maleficence. These principles have proved useful in addressing difficult medical cases. They're at the heart of a proper relationship between patient and family.

Autonomy

Autonomy relates to patients' ability to decide for themselves what level of care or intervention they want. Autonomy refers to an individual's ability (or substituted judgment by a surrogate) to choose but within certain limits and excluding irrationalities or acting against his or her own self-interest. Examples of exclusions include resuscitation or placing a tracheostomy or feeding tube to facilitate long-term care in a person who's already brain dead.

Neurosurgeons are perfectly justified in refusing to perform surgery on a patient who won't benefit from it, even if the patient or family members insist on trying everything. What are neuro-surgeons obligated to offer when families forcefully insist that "everything" be

COMMON BIOETHICS TERMS

Term	Explanation
Autonomy	Patient or family decides
Beneficence	Do what's best
Non-maleficence	Avoid doing harm
Justice	Fairness and all treated the same
Conflict of interest	Some other intention that has nothing to do with the illness
Coercion	Imposing your will on a patient
Paternalism	Doctor knows best and "don't tell me otherwise"

done? It's a challenging question, and answering it is particularly difficult when time is of the essence and it's not possible to have an independent expert do a comprehensive review. In this difficult spot, I think many surgeons respond by performing "Hail Mary" procedures.

Honoring an individual's autonomy requires the individual be fully capable of exercising it. Autonomy is closely linked to the ability to make a choice and to understand the condition and reasons for medical treatment. When an individual is comatose, autonomy is fully transferred to family members. Certainly, decision-making is simpler if an individual has previously drawn up an advance directive that details personal wishes or designates a relative to make those decisions.

There also are some patients who are inherently dependent on others and, thus, can't exercise autonomy. They defer to their significant other or offspring. Some people prefer the traditional model of deferring to the physician — "You're the doctor; you tell me." What we can't ignore is that we're all shaped by our relationships, which affect our choices and autonomy.

A major challenge to a patient's autonomy occurs if members of the health care staff use coercion in the form of manipulative language. An example would be strongly urging do-not-resuscitate orders or withdrawal of life support before the family is ready. In the United States, a physician shouldn't make a drastic change in an individual's care without the patient's or family's consent. In the rare instances in which it might be necessary to act, the reasons for doing so should be documented. The other extreme involves ignoring requests to reduce aggressiveness of care, despite a family signaling that they've had enough. It's important that physicians adopt a relational and sharing approach, and remain free of favoritism.

Justice

Another mainstay of ethics is justice, which relates to timeliness of care and full access, irrespective of age, insurance status, co-morbidity or lifestyle. With this principle, a patient with clearly self-inflicted comorbidities (such as coma after alcohol or drug intoxication or refusing to get vaccinated against SARS-CoV-2) should receive the same level of care as someone who's relatively healthy or whose illness isn't self-inflicted.

Resource rationing does occur daily in ICUs because some patients are sicker and the number of beds is finite. That's different, however, from withholding treatment based on a patient's prior behavior and lifestyle choices. Physicians aim to ration their time to balance the needs of each patient against other obligations, knowing that vulnerable members of the community must be protected, and discrimination, including presumed bias toward ethnically diverse populations, must be avoided.

Health care staff must practice utilitarianism, maximizing overall benefit, and providing equal service and opportunity to every individual. Physicians must avoid stereotyping, and inadvertently making an inappropriate remark is completely out of order. A moralizing stance is neither useful nor appropriate when interacting with an individual who may have made questionable choices.

Practicing justice means avoiding bias. In relationships, bias is an inclination for or against a certain group or individual. Uncorrected bias leads to prejudice and systematic negative treatment of people based on factors such as sex, race or ethnicity. By reflecting critically on our judgments, we avoid acting on harmful prejudice.

Bias, however, is everywhere, whether we recognize it or not. We may jump at the first available piece of information and "anchor" our decision-making process, even when the information is incorrect or changing. This can lead to poor decision-making.

With hindsight bias, we blame ourselves or others for not having anticipated certain outcomes, which might only be obvious now with the benefit of more knowledge. We also unfairly assume that other people share our experiences and have drawn the same conclusions. When a person is in a good mood, it's only natural to overestimate the likelihood of positive outcomes. Conversely, when someone is feeling down, it's more likely that he or she will expect negative outcomes. These personal emotions also drive irrational thinking.

TYPES OF BIAS THAT CAN AFFECT DISCUSSIONS ABOUT GOALS OF CARE

Bias	Explanation
Framing bias	Decision-making influenced by how the situation is explained and personal interpretation of medical information
Risk tolerance bias	Degree of willingness to accept a poor outcome
Regret bias	Avoidance of emotional pain associated with a decision that could result in a poor outcome
Alternative bias	Difficulty making decisions and a tendency to change preferences when many options are available

We as physicians need to guard against common biases. Part of our medical and nonmedical decorum is to practice ethics to the fullest by recognizing pitfalls, biases, and wrong choices and working them through.

Beneficence and non-maleficence

Beneficence, or beneficent care, generally means promoting good and withholding bad. "Of course!" one might say. But achieving beneficence requires the ability to empathize with the feelings, thoughts and attitudes of another person. Some health care staff come by this naturally, and for others, it must be learned. Empathy makes us curious about hidden emotional concerns in others and enables us to see the reality as another person perceives it. Many physicians view the concept of beneficence as the principle of improving quality of life, but it also involves the obligation to use medical knowledge appropriately.

Related to beneficence is non-maleficence, which simply means avoiding harm. Among comatose patients, practicing non-maleficence is not about avoiding prolonged suffering — individuals in a deep coma don't actually suffer. Rather, we seek to avoid unnecessary treatments that carry very serious adverse effects and could cause additional harm.

Families often ask why their loved one suddenly got worse when everything seemed to be heading in the right direction. Seemingly acceptable interventions (given the family's perception that the physician is doing all possible to change the situation) may actually be harmful. Examples include undergoing multiple brain surgeries, or continually withdrawing

INFORMED CONSENT

Until the 1970s, informed consent for procedures, let alone clinical studies, didn't exist or was undocumented. That changed after two watershed moments: the growth of medical bioethics as an academic specialty and passage of the American Hospital Association's 1973 Patient's Bill of Rights. The result of these advances is that patients can't be forced to proceed with anything in medicine.

Patient autonomy is closely linked to the ability to choose and understand the rationale and consequences for medical or surgical treatment. Individuals have the right not to participate in a study and the right to take time to make a well-reasoned decision. It's essential that there's no indication of coercion. The once universally accepted old tropes of "doctor knows best," "the fighting doctor" and "the doctor that never gives up" no longer apply.

and reinstituting a ventilator. Rather than being overt, harm to the patient may be subtle. For example, it may result from endless, overly aggressive treatments and surgical interventions that cause families to run up large medical bills.

OTHER CONCERNS

Beyond the four pillars are many other ethical issues health care staff deal with on a routine basis.

Confidentiality

Another facet of ethics is confidentiality. The patient or family members decide who can and can't be informed. However, because most individuals with an acute neurologic condition are unaware of their illness, disclosure of personal information to family members (or a surrogate) is necessary without a patient's consent. Nevertheless, confidentiality should still be preserved in the sense that patient information remains strictly on a "need-to-know" basis and should only be shared with health care staff directly involved in the individual's care.

Dignity

An important goal of ethics is to preserve and protect patient dignity. Ideally, that should override choices that conflict with autonomy. Families may make choices that would strip a person's dignity, such as asking for everything possible even though doing so would further degrade the patient's condition. In a comatose patient with major, potentially life-threatening medical complications, major surgery may fix the immediate problem without improving the overall outcome. In these situations, respecting dignity may be interpreted as a merciful end to suffering.

Families often summarize lack of dignity best when they say, "He doesn't want to live like a vegetable." We often hear this when a loved one is on a mechanical ventilator or being fed through a tube, or when the patient's facial features have changed so dramatically that the person is unrecognizable to family members. However, some caregivers are convinced that they can maintain a loved one's dignity and ensure that the individual doesn't feel like a burden to others; in their minds, it's just the right thing to do.

Cultural and religious appreciation

There's a growing need to appreciate an increasingly interconnected global world. I believe it's one of the most important issues of today. A patient and family members may come from a different culture or have a different religious background. This can introduce complex situations and make communication more difficult.

For example, emotional expressions vary within cultures, and what's acceptable in one may not be in another. Bereavement practices may differ. Views on when to withdraw life support may differ. All of these situations demand respect.

Because each faith tradition has its own rituals, opportunities for religious worship in the hospital should be provided, if requested by family members. Faith has a major effect on health care. It can serve as a coping strategy and offer hope of an afterlife and divine intervention that allows healing (not necessarily a cure).

Hope is a complex virtue (or vice). Many philosophers had something to say about hope. For philosopher Friedrich Nietzsche, hope was an illusion and a torment. For many people, hope is an optimistic attitude that keeps them going. Hope can turn to resignation when the time comes.

All faiths support preservation of life and avoidance of suffering, but some religious beliefs can be harmful if they prevent certain interventions or don't allow for withdrawal of care when care is incontrovertibly futile. Family members also may become resentful if they feel that their prayers for a loved one aren't answered. Families with a religious worldview may struggle with whether God has caused their pain.

Faith remains a personal matter for all — patient, family members and health care staff. Nobody should impose one's own values on others.

Prioritizing care

The fair-innings principle applies here. It advocates that every individual must have the same opportunity to experience all stages of life: childhood, young adulthood, middle age and old age. In cases when resources are limited, young people are generally put first because they've had the least opportunity thus far. Empirical evidence also suggests that most people believe that younger patients should receive priority. Physicians emphasize that among younger individuals ICU admission generally leads to a higher likelihood of survival and even a very acceptable outcome in some circumstances.

THE DECISION NOT TO RESUSCITATE

Do-not-resuscitate (DNR) orders are common. Despite having a DNR, many ICU patients receive aggressive care (and live to talk about it), and everyone in an ICU receives the best possible care.

There's a perception that the level of care received and DNR orders are inversely related, which may be true. In other words, a DNR could potentially lead to less attention from a physician and less aggressive care in individuals who are older and have prior serious illnesses. However, reasons for DNRs are broad, and DNRs shouldn't be taken out of context. DNR should not be initiated if there's a strong chance that the patient can turn around quickly after a medical intervention or if there's the possibility the initial neurologic examination isn't fully reliable.

Astute physicians are aware a CT scan of the brain may look very troublesome but understand the main determinant in considering DNR discussions should be a full clinical evaluation and comprehensive neurologic examination. We discourage early decisions (within hours of symptom onset) unless the clinical findings are obviously grim.

Also, it's important to understand that DNR involves both intubation and placement on the ventilator and restarting heart function. You cannot do one without the other. In the past, DNRs were reserved for patients who clearly were dying. Broader DNRs are relatively new in medicine, and specifically in critical care. Let me review how they've developed over time.

With the advent of ventilators to support patients with acute brain injury, physicians started questioning the advisability of using extraordinary procedures to maintain life in comatose patients. In the United States, these ethical discussions started in the 1970s, when the prominent physician Henry K. Beecher felt pity for the plight of families of comatose patients who didn't improve but were kept alive on a ventilator. He named it the "agonizing death watch" of the family. As an anesthesiologist, he encountered such patients daily and felt helpless to comfort nursing staff and families. His goal was to gain some closure for families.

Around the same time, Edwin (Ned) H. Cassem, a Jesuit priest and psychiatrist at Harvard Medical School, framed the dilemma in a different, more accusatory way: "Can the time come for terminally ill patients when medical treatment is a disguised form of abuse?" Neurosurgeons and neurologists were certain nothing would change, but worried they'd be held legally (and criminally) liable for removing a ventilator. And of course, hospital administrators on the sidelines wanted to avoid such unpleasant discussions. But we all understood that costly procedures in hopeless cases could and should be avoided.

Saving lives by way of "full court press" and "do everything you can, doctor" were mantras of the 1950s and 1960s. Medicine, and particularly intensive care medicine, was about providing the best care, delivered by the best-trained physicians, to maximize survival of a disorder that was spiraling out of control. Internist Mitchell T. Rabkin and his colleagues at Beth Israel Hospital clearly spelled out for the first time the criteria and circumstances when DNR orders would be appropriate.

Today, patients are resuscitated unless health care staff is explicitly directed otherwise. A DNR directive is justified when quality of life is anticipated to be very poor or when a severe disability or vegetative state is expected. Families frequently say that their loved one would not want to languish in a nursing home. What they mean isn't always clear (it varies a lot), but there's a sense that being totally dependent on others isn't an acceptable outcome. A few surveys conducted in ICUs suggest that few families want resuscitation in elderly debilitated patients.

A DNR order implies that cardiopulmonary resuscitation is withheld but all other treatment continues. Dr. Rabkin and colleagues clearly stated that given irreversible illness and imminent death, the appropriateness of cardiopulmonary resuscitation should be discussed and considered by a patient's physician. However, the individual and family members also had to weigh in.

DNRs were born out of a desire to bring transparency and clarity to an existing mishmash of approaches — such as "try it once" or "resuscitate but do not intubate" — and very often, private discussions among physicians that weren't always shared with a patient or family members or were quickly forgotten.

Other groups categorized ICU patients into multiple tiers of care, a categorization that still works very well and is easy to understand. New patients are automatically assigned to Category I: Use of all resuscitative efforts. Category II is for individuals with slim (but not impossible) chances of surviving, who continue to receive maximum therapy until health care staff become convinced that the prognosis is poor. These patients are treated aggressively for an additional 24 hours, and then the situation is reassessed. Category III is for patients whose estimated chances of survival are in the magnitude of 1 in 100,000. This designation requires consensus among physicians and nursing staff that further aggressive care is futile. Category IV is for patients who fulfill the clinical criteria of brain death, for whom "the conscious decision is made to relinquish a life which no longer has meaning," and indicates active withdrawal of mechanical ventilation.

In 1983, Dr. Rabkin and his colleagues discussed DNRs in a publication from the President's Commission for the Study of Ethical Problems in Medicine and Biomedical and Behavioral Research, called "Deciding to Forego Life Sustaining Treatment." The document defined levels of care as "heroic" or "ordinary," and tiers of treatment were categorized as "withholding" or "withdrawing."

The document underscores that there's no ethical difference between stopping therapy and failing to initiate therapy. The committee accepted that surrogates or proxies for a patient could express the patient's wishes for de-escalating care. In subsequent decades, additional sets of guidelines and position papers have followed.

We've achieved a new era in medicine, in which limitations on care can be justly applied to satisfy all those involved in caring for individuals who fail to thrive.

LETTING GO

When patients are in very poor health and don't improve, at some point, families, physicians and nursing staff realize that all that's being done is without any measurable goal. This often leads to what's called a "goals-of-care discussion." These conversations are necessary to summarize what's been done, the results, and what can reasonably be expected in the future. In my experience, it's often family members who first ask, "What are we doing here?"

Aside from the actual loss of someone you love and recognizing the finality of it, talking about letting go is very difficult and sometimes can cause a lot of pain. Messages from society often factor into this decision. They include:

- "Comfort care is basically giving up."
- "Cure happens because we fight back."
- "Intensive care physicians torment people they can't help."
- "The knowledge of medical professionals is God-given and not to be opposed by human action."
- "When there's medical futility, comfort care is the only compassionate option."

Disagreements about a topic as emotionally trying as withdrawing life support will likely never go away, and we can't expect everyone to view these situations in the same way. Quality of life is a vast topic. Physicians all over the world try to help patients and families in every imaginable way; however, there's no doubt that decisions concerning withdrawal of care are highly influenced by acute emotions.

Up to 20% of deaths in the United States each year occur in ICUs, many of them due to withdrawal of life support when nothing further can be done to benefit a patient. Practices for withdrawing life support — taking the patient off the ventilator and discontinuing medication — vary around the world. Some are more lenient, others are more restricted. Several European countries don't allow futile care; others have courts decide. In Asian and Middle Eastern countries, physicians practicing end-of-life medicine can experience considerable cultural pushback. However, those cultures are changing rapidly as younger physicians adopt Western values regarding the practice of medicine.

Ethicists have a more defined perspective regarding withdrawal of care. In the late 1980s, the Hastings Center published comprehensive ethical guidelines for end-of-life care. The guidelines focus on recognizing a patient's right to refuse unwanted life-sustaining treatment and propose a standard for surrogate decision-making. First, when an individual's wishes are known, they should be followed. Priority must be given to what a person wants. Second, when an individual is incapable of decision-making, we should rely on a proxy to decide, considering the patient's wishes and values. Third, absent information about those values, a decision should be made in accordance with a patient's best interests.

The Hastings Center guidelines also recommend using time-limited trials of treatment before making decisions — the "We tried but were unsuccessful" approach. The document also addresses the need to improve pain relief, recommends rejecting treatment requests that can't accomplish hoped-for objectives, and clearly separates withdrawal of treatment from physician-assisted suicide and euthanasia.

Advance directives can be helpful in making withdrawal-of-care decisions. An advance directive is a legal document signed by an individual when the person still has full mental capacity. The purpose of the document is to inform family members of personal preferences regarding care in the event of a catastrophic situation. However, advance directives aren't ideal. They're filled with legal language that can be difficult to interpret. Sometimes, an advance directive contains additional handwritten directions, such as "only short-term ventilator use" or "only short-term cardiac massage," without specifics.

An advance directive is unlikely to include clear statements about a neurologic condition, such as being persistently comatose or dependent on 24-hour nursing care. From my perspective, existence of an advance directive is an indication that the patient thought this through and was clearly afraid of receiving unnecessarily prolonged care when he or she couldn't voice an opinion. What often influences this decision is the wish not to be a continuous burden, financially or emotionally. That's why I regard advance directives as an indication not to continue with medical care that's not helping.

Some family members might disagree. They may dispute whether their loved one fully understood the advance directive or insist that their loved one receives aggressive care at all costs. Or they may believe that advance directives should only apply when the patient has lost all brain function. An advance directive often remains difficult to interpret for next of kin, certainly if they're seeing it for the first time and haven't had discussions with their loved ones regarding their wishes.

Instead of "Do Not Resuscitate" on advance directives, I would like to see a statement such as "Allow Natural Death."

Then, of course, we must work to make sure we all understand what that means. When medicine can no longer offer a decent quality of life, then it should at least offer a peaceful quality of death.

AND FINALLY

Most patients receiving only comfort care are already in the hospital, and the decision not to provide aggressive measures was likely made when they were admitted, or shortly thereafter. For some individuals, however, comfort care starts after they've been admitted to a nursing home and experienced a major complication.

Withdrawal of care from a comatose individual after several years of full support is highly uncommon, and such cases may reach the courts if there's a conflict between the physician and the family or between family members. This usually occurs when opposing sides take extreme positions and have irreconcilable views. The best-known U.S. cases have been those of Terri Schiavo and Karen Ann Quinlan. Media attention given to them created a political and legal circus.

Understand that this isn't the norm. In most situations, care is withdrawn when the family and the physician who most recently examined the patient agree that there's no opportunity for meaningful improvement. In instances where there are contentious issues, a member of a hospital or nursing home ethics commit-tee may be brought in to provide advisory adjudication and to try to keep the case from going to court.

How should health care providers and families interact?

CHAPTER 9

A CONVERSATION

Physician: I'd like to talk to you about where we're at with your brother and what we're finding worrisome. All the members of his health care team who've taken care of him are here plus our chaplain and social worker. We've invited them so that we can build a common understanding and all get on the same page.

Family: Our sister also is joining this meeting on speakerphone.

Physician: After we've introduced ourselves, I'll summarize your brother's condition and discuss issues with his health that are worrisome. Then let's talk about what matters most to him, what he's proud of doing and what he enjoys

most. Finally, I'd like to reach a consensus about what we're hoping for.

Family: Thank you for considering our needs.

The relationship between health care providers, a patient, and the patient's family has always been central in medicine. Ideally, this relationship embodies respect, compassion, integrity, trust and authenticity.

But these may be just empty words or could apply to any situation, if we don't consider what all of those concepts really mean. The same can be said of terms such as *the best care, excellence* and *professionalism.* Again and again, families will say that good communication with physicians is their most important need when a loved one has a neurocritical illness. Interaction with nurses, social workers and clergy also is vital.

THE PHYSICIAN-FAMILY RELATIONSHIP

The assumption in previous chapters is that a patient's family members and health care staff have a warm and compassionate relationship. That's essential, but family members of an individual who's comatose often are overwhelmed by a situation they never anticipated and feel vulnerable because of so many unknowns. Human nature also is distorted by biases and misconceptions, which often are hardwired in our brains and difficult to unlearn. But we shouldn't forget that most humans want to do good.

Entering an intensive care unit (ICU) is intimidating, particularly when a loved one's status is touch-and-go. Equally, health care staff of every stripe also are suddenly faced with a patient who has an acute, and often unique, problem that requires constant attention and decision-making. Staff must make rapid-fire decisions, sometimes more than 50 in one day. Our goal is always to get a patient through the immediate danger, whatever the cause of a coma and however grave the injury, while acknowledging the limitations of care.

Much has been written about the physician-patient and nurse-patient relationships and what patients and their families want. There are also informal codes of behavior for health care providers, most of which are common sense.

In the 19th century, Sir William Osler, possibly the world's greatest physician, wrote a magnum opus, *The Principles and Practice of Medicine*, which reformed medical education. He once remarked, "The profession of medicine is distinguished from all others by its singular beneficence." Physicians must commit to providing undivided attention and must recognize the expectations placed on them: to be trusted, confident, nonjudgmental and assertive. They should never pretend to be heroes, magicians, gods or members of a white-coated order of knighthood. Nor are they buddies, neighbors or chums. They'll always try to maintain some distance, despite being available for everything.

For families, a physician's ability to communicate is extremely important, and if those skills are poor, families may equate them with poor medical or surgical skills as well. Certainly, families don't want to deal with obnoxious, irritating physicians, even though they may be knowledgeable and highly skilled. At the same time, a physician who presents a medical opinion with a high degree of justifiable uncertainty — "Yes, recovery is possible, but I doubt it" — may confuse and frustrate family members.

Physicians also are aware that their behaviors and personal values can impair a cordial relationship. Whether they're naturally optimistic or pessimistic, they try to stick to the scientific (evidence-based) facts.

Over multiple conversations with a patient's family members, an attending physician has the not-insignificant burden of predicting how the patient will progress, the degree of disability, how the patient will look in 3 to 6 months or even a year, how many additional complications can be expected, and how well the patient may cope with additional medical issues, such as dialysis.

In truth, we seldom have all the answers because: 1) not every patient is the same; 2) comparisons are always difficult; 3) acute brain injuries generally are unpredictable; 4) there's considerable therapeutic uncertainty; and 5) prognosis often depends on a patient remaining stable, but it can change if the individual gets worse or develops complications.

Families want constant updates to relieve their anxiety. But it's not enough just to communicate with a patient's family. We must ensure that they understand what's happening to their loved one. I often close conferences by asking family members whether everything that was said made sense and what else they'd like to know. Personally, I'm a bit annoyed by books that describe how best to communicate with family members. I find some of the instructions (for example, "make eye contact," "check for understanding," and "recognize emotional cues") as mere common sense.

During conversations with family, it's important that physicians minimize their use of medical jargon. They shouldn't constantly ask you about understanding — "Can you tell me in your own words what I just told you?" — or repeatedly ask if you've been through something like this before. Some physicians also find it difficult to share emotions despite their best attempts to express genuine feelings of sympathy and distress about the situation a family is in.

Although physicians may need experience to elicit from family a patients' values and preferences, these skills come with time. I'm a strong proponent of building individual skill sets through trial and error, and it takes some stumbles and falls to get there. Self-help papers and books can easily overwhelm physicians with instructions on how to and how not to have a serious conversation.

Shared decision-making

The attending physician is the main medical decision-maker and is responsible for treating the patient. But decisions must (and this is a big must) also be made based on an individual's best interests, which is basically the individual's wishes and feelings about possibly living with major limitations.

This is where shared decision-making comes in. Families play a critical role in determining how long to extend life and how aggressively to provide treatment. They look for clues to a loved one's values and beliefs in several ways. They may recall comments that were made in the past after seeing someone in a similar situation ("If I'm ever on a ventilator, please don't let me live on"). They may revisit conversations they had with the patient ("Mom, what do you want me to do if you have a major stroke?"). Or they may have a document, such as a living will, that spells out requests regarding end-of-life care. Lacking such conversations or documentation, a family will have to consider whether their loved one thought about these issues, and what the person's responses might have been if asked.

Shared decision-making means a bit more than agreeing on a course of action. It may mean reaching a compromise, in essence, meeting in the middle. There are two unwelcome extremes — physicians who assert their prerogative to make the final decision and families who refuse to consider medical opinion. I view shared decision-making as finding the best option for the patient and getting to know what aspects of life that person valued.

It's important for family members to acknowledge that their personal views shouldn't take priority over their loved one's wishes. A family member may decline aggressive care ("This isn't what he would have wanted.") despite a potentially good prognosis with the likelihood of significant improvement over time. On the other hand, a patient may have clearly told family members "Do not let me go so easily." But now that their loved one is severely incapacitated and not doing well, honoring that request doesn't equate with what anyone would consider a state of well-being. It's important not only to distinguish between preference ("Do everything you can do") and value ("Don't let me live in a hopeless state") but also to consider the benefits, risks and perhaps even costs.

Avoiding conflict

Despite the good intentions of all parties, relationships between family members and the health care team can sour. Discussing the need for intensive care with families is difficult, particularly when family members are feuding or their worldviews don't align due to racial, religious or ethnic diversity. Some team members may be unsure how to balance cultural priorities, human needs and the seemingly endless medical possibilities.

It's not always clear why a breakdown in communication occurs. But professionals who behave inappropriately or carelessly or who display excessive pride or self-confidence should be called out because their behavior can exacerbate divisions. Letters of complaint from families often mention that a physician was bright and knowledgeable but also somewhat pompous. Frequent switching of services and doctors can disrupt communication and a patient's continuity of care.

Cultural issues also can be a barrier. In some cultures, directness is viewed as cruelty to the patient and perceived as doing more harm. In addition, some people may be less likely to trust a physician from a different race or ethnic group, particularly if there are language barriers. Differences in faith sometimes can become a barrier as well.

Finally, family structure and disagreement between family members about how to proceed in view of their loved one's preferences frequently lead to conflicts between families and health care providers.

Even previously close family relationships can be frayed by exhaustion and stress when a loved one is in the ICU for a long period of time.

Despite these issues, it's often possible to resolve conflicts between family members and health care providers. In my experience, taking time to talk with family members and to explain what we're seeing and doing for their loved one is immensely helpful. Physicians should always acknowledge hope when it exists, and so, too, realism when not much more can be done. Even in the worst scenarios, it's important for family to keep the lovely memories they have of their loved one.

Let me try to explain where we, as health care providers, are coming from. Then I'll describe the type of conversation and social interaction we want to have with a patient's family to achieve the most satisfactory outcome.

OVERVIEW OF HEALTH CARE TEAM

A member of the medical staff, as defined in federal regulations, is anyone authorized to provide medical care. In the ICU, that includes nurses, respiratory therapists, nurse practitioners, physician assistants, physicians, and individuals being trained in these specialties. In addition, there are ICU cardiologists, anesthesiologists, infectious disease experts, nephrologists and neuro-intensivists. Many modern ICUs have their own pharmacists, who participate in daily rounds to advise and document medication use.

Neurointensivists

Neurointensivists are doctors trained to deal with acute disorders of the brain and spine. They understand the deterioration that occurs after a major catastrophe. Neurointensivists also consult on other illnesses with neurologic concerns and possess core skills in interpreting neuro-imaging and other brainwave activity studies. Most often, a neurointensivist directs patient care in neuroscience ICUs.

Models of co-primary care also exist in which health care staff from two or more specialties are closely involved. For example, a patient with a traumatic brain injury who undergoes surgery to remove a clot will be cared for by neurosurgeons and neurointensivists. If complications occur, ICU infectious disease specialists and nephrologists may be consulted. Generally, the major task of a neuro-intensivist is to orchestrate a cohesive plan for assessing and managing a patient and preventing gaps in the patient's care.

Neurologists

Neurologists generally take a more "hands-on" role. They may look closely at a patient and yell at or shake an un-responsive individual in hope of eliciting a response. Neurologists may touch, pinch and continue to pinch (very hard) the person, again, hoping to achieve the desired response. They may probe a patient's body or superficially stick needles into the patient's skin. They may turn the person's head sideways to detect eye movement, shine a light into the eyes, touch a cornea with a tissue or a piece of cotton, or squirt water in an eye. Neurologists may move the patient's limbs back and forth to feel muscle tone.

In individuals who've recovered from a coma, neurologists look for actions that suggest unusual thought processes, such as repetition of a word, a changed mood, or an inability to concentrate on tasks or make simple decisions. Neurologists may test for memory retention, speech (understandability, slowness and slurring), reading and naming ability, vision, and hearing. Neurologists also may evaluate the stability of a person's stance and walk and use provocative tests, such as walking heel to toe and standing with the eyes closed.

Neurologists generally start with a general idea (a "working diagnosis") and then test and refine as they go along. They work on the balance of probability and carefully weigh all the data about a patient and, when necessary, review the data with another neurologist. Because findings on a neurological exam may fluctuate, another opinion can be helpful.

Neurosurgeons

Neurosurgeons are another primary contact. They make recommendations about whether the patient is an appropriate candidate for brain surgery. As I've discussed previously, surgery might involve removing a large portion of the skull to create more room for swelling, removing a tumor or a blood clot, or placing a drain. Many neurosurgeons also

practice what's known as interventional neuroradiology. This involves using a catheter instead of traditional surgery to remove clots from large brain arteries or injecting drugs into spasming arteries following a ruptured brain aneurysm.

Trauma surgeons

Trauma surgeons specialize in management of major trauma. They treat patients with head injuries but also individuals who have major injuries to the liver or spleen and bone fractures. Trauma surgeons often are called when a person has bleeding in the chest or belly. In situations in which a patient's life is in danger and there's trauma to the brain, a trauma surgeon typically consults with neurosurgeons and neurointensivists, assuming they're available at the hospital. Hospitals without a neurologist on call or a neurosurgeon at hand often will transfer a patient who's comatose to another hospital that can provide a higher level of care.

Nurses

Nurses in neurology ICUs are highly trained in the care of individuals with brain and spinal injuries. They administer drugs, monitor and alter infusions according to directives, maintain access to veins, closely monitor vital signs, and closely participate in resuscitation of patients in the event of a respiratory or cardiac arrest.

Neurology ICU nurses also educate family about the appearances and behaviors of patients and encourage families to be involved in the care of their loved ones. This helps family members to understand their loved one's condition and the complexity of care.

Nurses are trained in techniques for communicating with family members during times of significant stress who may not be familiar with medical terminology. They focus on maximizing the role of a patient's family rather than attempting to exert power and control over them. When a nurse forms a special connection with a patient, that can be comforting to the family.

Others

Social workers and chaplains also are part of the health care team. They're available soon after a patient is admitted. Social workers can help assess whether a patient will need long-term home care and identify resources if there's a problem with health insurance coverage.

The American College of Critical Care Medicine recommends that spiritual care be provided to patients and their families. In the United States, a clergy member's first encounter with a patient often is triggered by referral from health care staff or because it's hospital protocol. These professionals visit patients and provide them with moral support. If requested, they can offer anointing, blessings and prayer. Clergy can be essential to families at the time of a loved one's death and in the days that follow. Some families, however, prefer

not to have clergy present and even find it intrusive.

Teaching hospitals also have residents and fellows who see patients. They may be the first on the scene when something goes wrong. It's often residents who visit with family members following morning rounds to explain care plans for the patient. Medicine is very much a specialty of apprenticing. Multiple lines of communication can change plans, and that's not usual in complex situations.

THE FAMILY

Family members are part of the health care staff's social organization. Spouses and significant others are welcome as friends and confidants. The closer family members are to the patient, the more effective our discussions and conferences with them can be. If family members can't be present physically, we encourage them to participate by phone or online.

When I come to work and walk in the ICU, I see families strolling the hall, some on their phones giving updates to other family members. Many are in our family room, waiting to speak with a member of the health care team or for their loved one to return from a test or procedure. We get to know each other well over a period of days and weeks.

How much families know about coma and where they go to seek information varies. As we'll discuss in Chapter 10, families often turn to the internet for answers and to seek clarity on medical terms they read about or hear in conversation. When studied, more Google searches are carried out on the topic of brain death than on coma in general or coma recovery. One could argue this suggests a general unfamiliarity with the significance of brain death. Several websites provide information on rehabilitation after traumatic brain injury, whereas others offer support and an emotional outlet. Some, but not all, are reliable sources.

We don't always know how the families of our patients make decisions, but it appears that the patient's spouse often has the last word. Differences of opinion are common among family members of comatose patients, and sometimes these differences can lead to long-lasting conflicts. This is often the case when several people are involved, when emotions are high, and when the situation is extremely stressful.

The shaded box below lists some of the concerns that I've heard expressed by families as they try to make decisions regarding what's best for their loved ones.

Numerous surveys offer suggestions to help facilitate communication and improve family satisfaction concerning the care a loved one is receiving. These steps include:
- Family-support coordinators to improve communication between physicians and families
- Increased communication with doctors
- More-flexible visiting hours
- Family participation in morning rounds
- Separate hospital rooms to stay the night and to gather together
- Support groups
- Other types of resources

I've found what's most important is an open line of communication with families and frequent interactions with them. Even when that's achieved, the experience of spending time in an ICU still can be stressful for a family.

Care of family members

Having a loved one in a coma can affect the health of family members. Health

---

CONCERNS EXPRESSED BY FAMILY MEMBERS

- Not everyone in our family is on the same page. We don't agree.
- We don't want our loved one to suffer when dying.
- We don't want our loved one kept alive and severely disabled.
- Does this conflict with our religious beliefs?
- We're seriously concerned whether we can afford long-term care.
- We're not certain we know how our loved one will do over time.
- We don't know how to make such important decisions.

care staff also evaluate the well-being of family members, looking for indications of depression and anxiety. Family members may express an inability to cope with current circumstances. Some may voice feelings of being abandoned or punished by God.

A doctor or other member of the health care team may ask family members what typically brings them strength and comfort, and whether they're interested in talking with a hospital chaplain. Chaplains provide spiritual care, usually regardless of a family's beliefs and practices. A chaplain's straightforward approach to asking simple questions about religion is very important and may be appreciated when family members are struggling.

WHERE WE MEET

Where we talk with families is almost as important as what we discuss and how we express it. Obviously, we can't have a serious conversation in a hallway or another busy part of the hospital. Some ICUs include a gathering space where families can talk, reflect and rest. Many modern ICUs have rooms especially designed for family conferences. We also speak to families personally at the bedside, but if there are a lot of people, we'll use a large conference room.

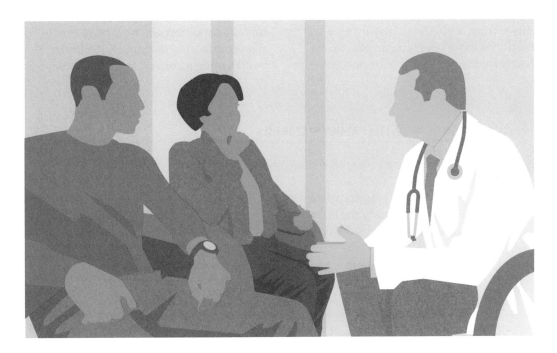

Meetings with family may involve a private conversation with the closest family members or a larger gathering with extended family.

The first of these personal meetings usually happens when an individual is admitted. The goal is to communicate the person's condition on arrival, what plans are in place and whether emergency surgery is needed. These meetings are emotionally charged, and family members may not grasp everything they're being told. I follow up regularly if the patient's situation is constantly changing or when a new development occurs. Larger, all-inclusive group meetings or conferences come later, at which point the health care team reassesses the situation and sets goals of care for the coming weeks.

A meeting at the bedside allows us to show things to family members that will help them understand why their loved one reacts (or doesn't) in a certain way. In this setting, a physician may involve family members in trying to elicit a response from the patient or demonstrate what a certain response, such as squeezing a hand, means. We can confirm what family has witnessed or explain that some responses are reflexive and not voluntary. (As I noted in Chapter 1, spontaneous grimacing, yawning, and tearing are often involuntary responses that may be confusing to families.)

Failure to focus or fixating on objects is an important finding that can be shown to family members. We also can point out other complications. When a patient awakes from coma and is attentive, plans for further rehabilitation are discussed with family members at the bedside.

Every time they enter a patient's room, physicians must be prepared to update family members about their loved one's current condition and may need to answer lingering questions. We try to avoid having a conversation in a patient's

CONVERSATIONS WITH FAMILY MEMBERS

- Gather all close family members, nursing staff, clergy, social workers, and other medical providers.
- Have all relevant test results available.
- Have one person (usually the attending staff physician) lead the conversation.
- Identify the person who is most responsible for decisions.
- Discuss the patient's current state, management and complications.
- Discuss whether the patient is aware of his or her condition.
- Discuss the current care plan.
- Discuss care options.
- Discuss the expected timeline for improvement or possible point of no return.
- Discuss code status and resuscitation efforts.
- Schedule a follow-up meeting.

room with people on cellphones asking questions. Families also need to understand that physicians in other specialties may come in and out of their loved one's room, and these experts will not want to answer questions outside their purview.

FAMILY CONFERENCES

A few ground rules often increase the satisfaction of everyone who attends a larger family conference. We often start by introducing the participants and explaining the purpose and process of the meeting. Larger conference rooms allow us to include more family members or close friends, and we always invite social workers, clergy, nursing staff and other specialists involved with a patient's care. These meetings are to provide information about the patient's current state, the level of care the person is currently receiving, and whether adjustments should be made.

Every attempt should be made to describe the patient's clinical condition unambiguously, especially with the closest family members. When appropriate, family members should be encouraged to meet face-to-face with the clinical staff. Information about the individual's clinical neurologic state should be expressed clearly. Having family members view the injury on a CT scan or MRI also can be helpful and may clarify the gravity of the situation.

It's important to discuss other issues that may be worrying family, such as the their loved one's experience of pain, why their loved one appears to be fighting the ventilator, the meaning of facial and limb twitching, and the cause of agitation.

I've found that ambiguous phrases such as "survive but disabled," "two-thirds will do poorly" or "cannot tell" often aren't helpful to family members. It's also my belief that in more dire situations the phrase "withdrawal of care" should be avoided. The message should be that everything is being done for their loved one, but the current care plan does not include aggressive care or interruption of the dying process.

In early conversations, physicians also try to discern a patient's wishes by asking questions or making statements, such as: "If your loved one was sitting here, what would he or she think?" or "What did your loved one value the most, and what would dramatically impact his or her daily joy and satisfaction?"

During such conversations, families often will grieve and cry, and appropriate silences are often necessary. Sometimes, these larger conversations may lead to a decision to withdraw critical care and move to comfort measures. Some family members are prepared and fully understand what is ahead and what their loved one wants. Many need some time to adjust, particularly if what happened was totally unanticipated.

I've found that after a family decides to withdraw care, the mood often changes, and family members come to terms rather quickly with their decision. I've seen sadness quickly turn to relief. In cases when family relationships have been fractured, mending may begin. A follow-up meeting may be necessary, and if possible, it should take place later the same day or the next day, when other family members have arrived or the situation has been discussed with them in detail.

In short, as family members ricochet between hope, despair and acceptance, they appreciate knowing their loved one's physician remains involved on the sidelines and can be called upon when needed.

The facts and the truth

The practice of medicine — in particular neurology — are based on two major guiding principles: skepticism and self-inspection. When physicians examine and care for a patient, we're naturally full of doubt about what we've found. We constantly question whether what we did was correct, given what we see on an examination. We're always asking ourselves whether we could have done something differently. My motto, shared by many of my colleagues, is "I doubt it." We need to find facts because facts lead to truth and transparency.

At the same time, we can't and shouldn't hide anything from family members, even if the news isn't good. Of course, physicians should be allowed to explain comprehensively to families why care is futile. I think many of us would agree that providing futile care could actually harm a patient because no treatment is

without risks. Providing unlimited care presents major ethical challenges, and the financial costs are substantial. Doing everything can be wrong in certain circumstances, and it's important to have a conversation about that delicate topic.

Conflicts

I'd be remiss if I didn't say that not all family conferences go well. The dynamics between physicians and family members vary, and strong opinions, especially those expressed or held before a conference even begins, can lead to unsatisfactory outcomes.

Strong opinions from family members, and sometimes physicians, may be factors. Some physicians believe that poor outcomes occur from "calling it quits too soon," resulting in a self-fulfilling prophecy; the outcome is bad because we didn't do enough. They think other physicians give up too often and too early. These physicians remain hopeful despite all odds and always see a silver lining in bad news. Sometimes, though not often, physicians believe that the "sanctity of life" trumps everything, and they don't want to be involved in any action that leads to early withdrawal of support. When a family has strong conflicts with the attending physician, it may be time to hand over the care of the patient to someone else who's willing to consider all options.

When an individual doesn't awaken and CT scans confirm devastating brain damage, some physicians still think they see signs of improvement each day. They often focus on details of daily care and not on prognosis. Some physicians simply don't wish to confront the issue of withdrawing care, while others are more comfortable doing so. Physicians also may ask colleagues for advice, which can render differing opinions. Discussions about a patient may go in many different directions, and decisions may come quickly or not at all, or the patient may receive care without any reflection on whether it's actually helping.

AND FINALLY

Neurology and neurocritical care are learned by examining patients, talking to their families, and being at the bedside, as often and as long as needed. They're not learned just from reading textbooks.

Most physicians in these specialties work quietly behind the scenes of the hustle and bustle of an ICU. Among themselves, they often discuss options, best goals of care, how interactions went, and how to resolve differences of opinion.

The goal is to create an environment of trust and care. Patients should always have a physician's best attention and nothing less. This philosophy is an underlying theme of this book, which seeks to provide families with insight into a fully unexpected, initially tragic situation.

Many physicians recognize their own limitations. We're never rewarded for what we could avoid and are more often challenged for what we missed. Daniela Lamas, a pulmonology and critical care physician wrote in the *New England Journal of Medicine*, "In contrast to the protocols we follow for much of critical care, our approach to communication with surrogate decision-makers (family), though well intentioned, is often haphazard and unsupportive."

We always strive to improve our interactions with families. That includes training in effective communication and carefully explaining to families what we know, and what we don't know. We meet with families as soon as possible after their loved one is admitted and confer with them regularly thereafter. Our best efforts, however, may not always reduce the stress on family members or increase their satisfaction with the care their loved one is receiving. We have a long way to go in that regard.

What about experimental and unproven therapies?

CHAPTER 10

A CONVERSATION

Physician: I understand that you'd like my opinion on new treatments you've read about. I'd be happy to share my views.

Family: We appreciate that. We read on the internet that some centers are saying that they can cure coma. They're saying patients they've treated have woken up after months or even years. But our insurance won't cover that type of care, and we don't know if it's worth the effort and money.

Physician: It's important to put the information you've read into perspective. We're committed to helping your daughter, but I'm sure you wouldn't want her to be harmed or to receive unnecessary treatments.

Family: You're right, but we've heard some good things about stimulation and music therapies. And what about stem cell therapy?

Families of comatose patients want to know that their loved one's physicians are doing all they can. Sometimes, though, that doesn't seem like enough, and family members may look to experimental and unproven treatments for solace.

The sheer volume of medical information about coma treatments is confusing, to say the least. It's hard to keep up with all the competing claims for different therapies, many of which are unknown to neurologists and neurosurgeons. Obviously, we're very careful about interpreting websites that include stories of people who supposedly used a particular product and then markedly improved. Often, these websites show before and after images of the patient in intensive care with nightmarish facial swelling, drains and bandages, and then smiling, triumphant and recovered years later.

These claims of remarkable recoveries have mushroomed all over the internet and on social media sites. This creates uneasiness among family members who are facing what, to them, seems to be the same set of circumstances. The physicians they talk to in the hospital seem to paint a much gloomier picture than what they're seeing online.

Many websites discuss conventional medical treatments and interventions for comatose patients. But other websites are dedicated to formidable claims for new, "exciting" treatments that are supported, at best, by half-truths. In other words, these treatments are presented without a meaningful explanation of how they could be helpful. Examples include music therapy, extensive physical therapy, active-awakening programs, magnetism, acupressure and acupuncture. And let's not forget vitamins, minerals, and even fish oil. There also are more-invasive therapies, such as low-intensity ultrasound pulsation and electronic lead implantations focused on areas of the brain such as the thalamus. (See Chapter 1 for more on the thalamus.)

Family members often ask me about stimulation therapies, stem cells, oxygen therapy, and even brain transplantation.

Such questions are understandable if a loved one's progress has stalled, the improvement is minimal, or there seems to be one complication after another.

Family conferences to discuss goals of care often are the best setting in which to discuss both medically sound and unproven options for treatment.

SORTING FACT FROM FICTION

Allow me to frame the current status of known treatment options. I'll try to explain what works and what doesn't, based on research. It would be a mistake however, to presume that research — even the latest studies — can provide answers to all the questions regarding treatment.

Let's start by reviewing some data. First, most individuals who are comatose awaken. And virtually all individuals who awaken from a coma due to an acute brain injury — not just those due to a drug overdose — don't remember their time in the ICU or even a large part of their hospital stay. They have no recollection of how the days passed, whom they met, who took care of them, which tests they underwent, how many times they were poked with needles, or how often they were in surgery.

All of this proves that, fortunately, there are no long-lasting, traumatic after-effects from this experience. It doesn't exclude the possibility that patients who are starting to awaken from coma may be in a "twilight zone" where they retain select memories of events. Most of these individuals recover rapidly. Unfortunately, we have no way to test them to identify which specific treatments led to the good outcomes.

Second, in the acute phase of coma after necessary interventions, we have few treatment options. The best therapy is to have the brain heal itself and to act quickly when complications arise. (For example, swelling of the brain and increased pressure underneath the skull can cause a patient to lose all brain function.)

As highlighted in many parts of this book, if we give an individual time to recover and optimize care with aggressive support and treatment of complications, it's very likely that the person's eyes will open and he or she will become alert. This improvement may coincide with a recently introduced treatment, but it's far from clear whether there's a cause-and-effect relationship between the two events. Physicians withhold judgment on this point because we can't be absolutely certain that a patient wouldn't have awakened even without treatment.

I can honestly state that we can't reverse coma if we don't understand exactly how the interventions work. If we don't have solid scientific proof of a treatment's efficacy, we shouldn't be using it. In clinical science, it's not unusual that treatments accomplish a goal but also result in complications that negate all their positive effects. Many people have heard the expression "The cure is worse than the disease," and we've seen pharmaceutical ads on TV that show

symptom-free people enjoying leisure activities while an announcer in voiceover warns, "Don't take this medication if you have ... ." Moreover, experimentation can be dangerous for a patient and costly for families who believe the hype and are lured into expensive programs.

Another major issue is how people learn about coma and what they hear, aside from what's on the internet. Most people know that movies and TV shows aren't accurate reflections of reality. Nevertheless, information in the media about coma may still have a substantial influence. In a constantly changing news cycle and entertainment industry, there are many ways to tell a story, and airtime doesn't guarantee accuracy. And science itself often isn't good enough. It's appropriate to ask what to believe. Here is my assessment.

Coma in the media

What do you picture when you hear that someone is comatose? It's likely an image you saw on TV or the internet. Maybe it's a video you saw on social media. Are these image portrayals accurate? Do they only show miraculous cases? Who are the physicians in the media attempting to explain coma? All things considered, I'd advise a lot of caution and a healthy bit of suspicion concerning coma-based media rhetoric.

Broadly, the term *media* references the main sources of mass communication: broadcasting, publishing and the internet. The actor Neil Patrick Harris (*Doogie*

Howser, M.D.) once famously said, "I'm not a doctor, but I was paid to be one on TV." We might say the same for some doctors who are paid to be experts. The media often responds to medical stories as news items, and each network hires several "doctors" with variable backgrounds to comment on medical news, often outside their fields of expertise. Should we listen to them? Less astute medical experts on TV may be inclined to hasty judgments, lazy thinking and misinterpretations. Some seem genuinely astonished about cases most neurologists easily recognize as a diagnostic error.

For example, after reading about near-death cases over the years, I have an inkling that many involve hypothermia. That is, the person had a body temperature around 21 C and appeared to be dead until awakening after rewarming. In other patients, large amounts of sedative drugs may have taken longer than anticipated to clear from their systems. Then, after being pronounced irrecoverably comatose, they sat up in bed and chatted with visitors. These aren't miracles but rather failures to recognize major pitfalls and traps.

Some medical experts on TV lose the general context of the issue at hand and try to explain the inexplicable. Others may present information as incontrovertible evidence without opportunity for a response. What I know is that accounts about comatose patients with dramatic improvements often are biased toward the fantastic. What I hear about coma, vegetative state and brain death on TV is often risky, misleading and inaccurate information.

Deviations from reality

Many articles about coma on pop-culture websites or even in mainstream news sites are disturbing, and people may find it difficult to ferret out medical facts, especially when they're exposed to headlines suggesting that patients are more aware than expected. A common theme in media coverage of coma is that physicians had no hope for a comatose patient, but the family disagreed or there was disagreement among the family members about withdrawing support. Readers are left with an impression that differs markedly from the reality in the hospital.

Recovery from coma is rarely breaking news. Occasionally, dignitaries and survivors of a catastrophe, such as a major traffic accident, may get media attention. I reviewed newspaper articles about coma to see if the headlines and stories emphasized certain circumstances of the condition and provided a balanced view of expectations about awakening. I also wanted to see if articles accurately portrayed outcomes for given situations and how they described the sentiments of patients' family members and the decisions and judgments that were made about the comatose individual. It's not surprising that coma associated with acute injury was the most common theme in the news stories.

Reporters are often drawn to the tragedy of a young person with a sudden, catastrophic injury that led to a coma. However, the news reports I read tended to be skewed toward patients with a much higher probability of recovery and effective rehabilitation. A vegetative state was rarely a subject of interest and generally addressed only when a family or physician conflict emerged, or the case involved a miracle "awakening." When I closely read these articles, it appeared that none of the patients described were actually in a vegetative state.

Perhaps the most important inaccuracy in news reporting on coma was a failure to mention the role of medication in producing the coma. Only after I carefully read entire articles did I determine the patient was in a medically induced coma. Finally, most stories involved young individuals who had experienced violence or trauma. However, in U.S. hospitals, the average coma patient is approximately 60 years old.

Catchy headlines may grab people's attention, but communication psychologists have found that nuances in wording can change the way people read an article and what they remember about it. While most families recognize that news accounts about coma may be inaccurate, the stories still come up in our family conferences. Certainly, not all news media sensationalize medical news, but it's important to understand that medical stories reported in the news may not provide the complete story.

The internet

The internet has become a vital and increasingly convenient source for medical information. It's not uncommon for patients and families to consult the internet for help with medical decision-making when an acute situation arises. Research shows nearly 80% of internet users have searched for health information, making it the third most popular online activity. Family members often turn to the internet to seek clarification of medical terminology, learn more about a condition and search for the latest medical treatments. The accuracy and reliability of health information on the internet varies greatly.

With more than 1 billion users, YouTube is one of the largest platforms on the internet. Many families access YouTube to gather information about possible treatment options. Many videos about coma are available on YouTube. One study specifically looked at the reliability of such information and, in particular, at the association between brain death and organ donation. Organ donation was universally discussed in a negative light, and several sites accused physicians of falsely declaring someone dead to acquire organs. It's easy to see how coverage like that could negatively impact a family's perception of a physician's intent to declare someone brain-dead. Moreover, the same study showed that there was an abundance of false information, regarding the terms *brain death*, *persistent vegetative state* and *coma*, which were often used interchangeably.

I don't mean to imply that there are no reliable sources online because that's untrue. Monthly journals produced by professional organizations provide in-depth coverage of medical conditions including coma. For example, *Neurology Today* is the official publication of the American Academy of Neurology, and the editors are practicing neurologists. Also, every top-rated medical center in the United States has a website with medical information, as do the various centers and institutes that are part of the National Institutes of Health.

TV shows and movies

The general public's understanding of medicine, and particularly coma, often comes from TV shows and movies. A recent review of soap operas found that the recovery rate from coma they presented was unrealistic. Patients in two-week comas almost always made a full recovery, which is very different from what we see in clinical practice.

Some studies have examined how medical TV shows such as *House* and *Grey's Anatomy* introduce the topics of diagnosis, ethics and teamwork. By any criterion, the quality is very low. The episode "Son of a Coma Guy" in the celebrated series *House* is a case in point, with a bewildering mix of seizures from a genetic disease, vegetative state, transient awakening after medication and even a heart transplant.

Many movies also offer a dishonest view of the mystery of coma. It's a useful plot device for screenwriters, who show actors in a dream-like state having nightmares. The characters often experience personality changes and go on to recover and take revenge on the

person who put them in the coma. And families are greatly relieved when the person in a coma awakes against all odds.

Not surprisingly, movies that include an actor in a coma usually are thrillers involving motor vehicle accidents, gunshot wounds or violence that leads to the brain injury. Seldom do such movies shape information about a coma in a useful way or correctly convey to the public the major consequences of the condition and rehabilitation. In only a few instances is there an admirable combination of reportage and essay.

In the movies I've seen, actors portraying patients who were comatose for months weren't tracheotomized nor did they have contractures. None had feeding tubes. Most remained perfectly groomed, tanned and with good muscle tone throughout the coma, which trivializes the depiction of prolonged coma as a sleep-like state, such as with Sleeping Beauty. Sudden awakening from a coma occurred in nearly two-thirds of the actors and followed a characteristic pattern. The person was in a coma for several years, awakened within seconds as if from a terrifying nightmare, and was perfectly fine.

Of course, screenwriters or directors working in a genre other than documentary have no moral obligation to present factual representations. They can deviate from reality in fictional films to produce a certain desired effect to entertain. In a study we did in 2006, I asked viewers who watched film scenes depicting coma if they agreed or disagreed with this statement: "If my family member were in the same situation, it's possible that I'd remember what happened in the scene and allow it to influence any decisions that I'd make." Much to my surprise, roughly 1 out of 3 said yes. That hints at how much influence movies can have.

Audiences may be perceptive about news media and film approaches, but it's still difficult for viewers to know where to draw the line. Authors Gabrielle Samuel and Jenny Kitzinger summarized it as follows: "Be careful with terminology and metaphors; ... beware of making inappropriate comparisons (e.g., with short-term coma experiences); consider the potentially misleading power of images; ... reflect on the wider social context in which technologies will (or will not) be made available; and seek out a wider range of comment (including accessing the perspectives of patients, carers, and families where possible)."

CLINICAL STUDIES

Labels like *untested* and *unproven* get bandied about in conversations about coma treatments. They refer to evidence from clinical studies. *Untested* means that a therapy hasn't been investigated. Something untested also is *unproven*. Because of lack of testing and proof, *unsure* is where we're at with almost everything about coma. Allow me to briefly explain what evidence means in regard to studies of medical interventions.

First, we look at the design of the research to see if it applies to a given situation in

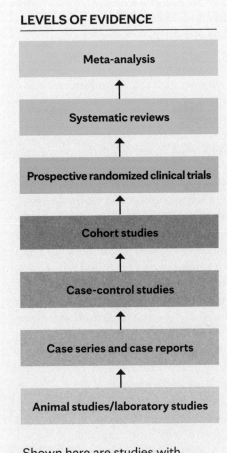

LEVELS OF EVIDENCE

Meta-analysis

↑

Systematic reviews

↑

Prospective randomized clinical trials

↑

Cohort studies

↑

Case-control studies

↑

Case series and case reports

↑

Animal studies/laboratory studies

Shown here are studies with different levels of evidence — from unknown or little importance on the bottom to best evidence at the top. In a case-control study, patients are compared with others in similar situations. In cohort studies, many patients are followed over time to determine their outcomes and risk for a condition or a disease. In clinical trials, participants are randomly assigned to receive an investigative therapy.

medicine and then we check what kind of study it is. There are several different levels of evidence in science (see the chart on page 173). The best evidence comes from well-designed clinical trials in which patients are randomized and neither the patients nor the investigators know which participants are receiving the investigative drug and which are receiving an inactive substance (placebo).

In this type of research, the distribution of known and unknown factors is the same among participants who are being treated (intervention group) or untreated (control group). Many patients are needed for a randomized controlled trial to ensure that the results will be valid. Randomized controlled trials are the gold standard in medical research. If a lot of randomized control trials are done involving the same treatment, the results can be pooled and assessed in a systematic review or meta-analysis.

It's more difficult to perform clinical trials for rare diseases or conditions. And the discouraging news is that none of the published studies about coma has produced strong data. Numerous test-tube, culture and animal studies have investigated interventions proposed to treat various types of acute brain injury. To date, however, no rigorous, well-designed clinical study has shown that any of the drugs or substances tested change the effects of acute brain injury. The only *possibly* helpful methods are neurocritical care and neurosurgery when feasible.

Quite often, potentially promising therapies get their start in a research

laboratory, and then they're tested in hospitals or clinics. Whether results from the lab can be transferred to the bedside is a common concern in medicine. This is partly because some animal experiments are poorly designed, and that leads to less success when a human clinical trial is done. Plus, humans don't always respond to treatment in the same way as laboratory mice or primates.

The former director of the Centers for Disease Control and Prevention, Thomas R. Frieden, summarized it well in 2017: "This 'dark matter' of clinical medicine leaves practitioners with large information gaps for most conditions and increases reliance on past practices and clinical lore." Families should be well informed about the nature of a clinical trial before signing up. They also should have a healthy suspicion about trials or experiments that aren't endorsed by major academic centers or run by experienced clinical investigators.

DRUG TREATMENTS

Solid data about drug treatments for coma are critical and lacking. The good news is that some brain-stimulating medications may help a patient who has emerged from a deep coma into a minimally conscious state. There are two major pathways in the brain that can be targeted with these medications: serotonin secretion and dopamine secretion. Antidepressants that selectively inhibit serotonin may benefit someone who is depressed and struggling after recovering from coma.

Dopamine is an important neurotransmitter that motivates people to take actions. Drugs that stimulate release of dopamine, particularly amantadine, have been used to treat individuals with traumatic brain injury. The authors of one amantadine study claimed that patients treated with the drug emerged from a coma more quickly after a traumatic brain injury. Unfortunately, the results have never been replicated in other studies or in situations outside of trauma.

The long-term effects of amantadine are unknown, and that's a critical piece of information. Giving serotonin inhibitors and dopamine stimulators to patients with traumatic brain injuries is "off label." That means their use in that setting hasn't been approved by the Food and Drug Administration (FDA) because there's insufficient proof that it will work.

The drug zolpidem is on investigators' radar screens because of some evidence that it makes individuals in a minimally conscious state more agitated and, thus, more awake. However, the drug often does the opposite and causes sleep, which is the use for which it was originally approved.

Some researchers have theorized that a cocktail of multiple drugs, including naltrexone, carbidopa-levodopa, donepezil, bromocriptine, modafinil, zolpidem, amantadine and dextroamphetamine, arouses neurotransmitters that have gone silent or stimulates neurons that are markedly deprived of natural substances. Using multiple medications at the same time makes it difficult to determine which ones are having an impact, particularly if they're being administered by someone who strongly believes in the treatment.

Some programs also have used vitamins, antioxidants, and immunonutrition to treat comatose individuals. We've found no credible evidence that any of these interventions help or harm patients. We also don't know if claims about benefits of stimulant medications will hold up in the long term, but the general impression is that they won't.

Sensory-stimulation programs

Sensory-stimulation programs often place a major burden on family members of comatose patients with little proven benefit. For up to eight hours a day, seven days a week, family members are asked to vigorously stimulate their loved one's skin and make sounds and loud noises at the bedside. The theory is that doing all this will make it more likely that a person will awaken.

Some sensory-stimulation programs also claim to reduce further breakdown of brain cells by keeping the cells constantly activated — the "use it or lose it" principle. However, these programs may produce sensory overstimulation — an admittedly difficult-to-define term — which actually produces the opposite effect of making their loved ones more tired. This is the reason why many hospital intensive care units control the number of patient visits and keep them short.

Music therapy also has been studied in comatose patients on the belief that music activates emotional functions in the brain and encourages arousal following brain trauma. Allegedly, physiological changes have been noted in these individuals during music therapy sessions, and it's been suggested that the program can be tailored to personal needs.

In some programs, a music therapist sings to a patient at the same pace as his or her pulse and in time with his or her breathing. A range of reactions has been observed in these studies from slower and deeper breathing to fine motor movements, hand grabbing, head turning, and eye opening to fully regaining consciousness. Patients in a vegetative state blink their eyes more in response to music than during silence, which investigators also attributed to increased arousal.

When the therapist first begins to sing, a patient's heart rate initially slows and then rises rapidly, sustaining an elevated level until the end of the contact. An EEG shows calmer brain rhythms. These reactions have been loosely interpreted as brain processing. The effect fades out, however, after the music stops. Other studies have suggested some stimulation with nature sounds, including blood pressure and heart rate improvements, as well as possible shortening of the duration of coma.

Unfortunately, none of the stimulation programs I've described supports a meaningful physiologic mechanism. There also isn't one well-designed, respected study showing that patients exposed to such stimulation awaken at all or more quickly than we'd expect based on their types of brain injuries. Some families bring in personal playlists for their loved ones, hoping the music can help shake their loved ones from their current states.

Other dubious claims

Placement of a drain in the brain's ventricles to reduce brain pressure in a comatose patient isn't uncommon, particularly if those fluid chambers have been widening. However, when someone is in a persistent vegetative state, the brain continues to shrink, and pressure isn't of any concern. In that case, placement of a tube connecting fluid chambers in the brain to a fluid compartment in the belly (a ventriculoperitoneal drain) may lower the patient's intracranial pressure, which could be harmful.

Sudden pressure changes that tug the brain down may cause clot formation between the skull and the brain. A ventriculoperitoneal drain, a last resort measure to improve coma, assumes widening of the ventricles is the main culprit, and it's always unsuccessful.

An often-suggested treatment for coma involves providing an individual with 100% oxygen at high atmospheric pressures to improve oxygen availability in the body (hyperbaric oxygen). Hyperbaric oxygen therapy (HBOT), involves breathing pure oxygen in a pressurized environment. It has been studied for traumatic brain injury. Supposedly, HBOT improves oxygen supply to an injured brain and reduces swelling associated with low oxygen levels. Unfortunately, adding more oxygen to the body isn't helpful if a cell is injured to the point that it can't absorb oxygen.

With HBOT, an individual is placed in an airtight chamber, the pressure within the chamber is increased, and the person is given 100% oxygen to inhale, which increases oxygen pressure in body tissues. The potential adverse effects of HBOT include damage to the ears, sinuses, and lungs from the increased pressure and oxygen poisoning. Therefore, benefits and risks of the therapy need to be carefully evaluated.

In cases of traumatic brain injury, there's little evidence that patients receiving HBOT have a good outcome. However, laboratory research shows that HBOT can reduce the severity of brain damage in comatose individuals after a cardiac arrest if the therapy is administered within two hours after the injury.

Results with HBOT in preclinical and clinical studies differ, and the crucial factor seems to be how long after an injury it's used. In clinical research, the earliest treatment is given six hours after an injury. However, 12 hours or longer is more common, which is much longer than has been done in laboratory (animal) research.

The bottom line is that we don't have enough evidence to determine whether HBOT is effective for individuals who are comatose after an acute brain injury.

A more aggressive treatment involves placing an electrode deep inside the brain to stimulate the thalamus. (The thalamus is basically a switchboard for signals going to the thinking and executive parts of the brain, as explained in Chapter 1.) These implants haven't been tested rigorously, and none of the patients in a vegetative state who've received it has recovered. One of those was Terri Schiavo, who became well known during her famous right-to-die legal case.

Whether the cells that "rev up" a person's alertness can be electrically stimulated remains an open question, although we know that neurons fire after triggering by electrical currents and chemical signals. Electrode implantation is tantamount to adding more battery power to a defective computer and not the equivalent of a soldering iron. Also, focusing on just one aspect of brain activity isn't enough because many parts need to function together to produce wakefulness.

Magnetic and transcranial ultrasound stimulation are other therapies that have been suggested. We don't know whether either would help patients or cause additional damage. Spinal stimulation and transcranial magnetic stimulation are also questionable. One study involved placing wires in the spinal cords of 200 patients in a vegetative state to stimulate their spines.

The investigators labeled the responses in more than half of the individuals as "excellent" or "positive." But the investigators' descriptions of the responses were ambiguous, such as "reaction toward various stimuli is rich emotional expression," "opening and closing eyes when a specific stimulus is detected," and swallowing when food was placed in mouth." The authors said the patients also had increased brain blood flow in the brain's frontal cortex, which controls executive functions. A randomized, controlled trial of dorsal column stimulation was proposed but hasn't been performed.

Transcranial magnetic stimulation produced similar results in another study. While all these preliminary clinical results have been called "intriguing and encouraging," they are nothing more than that.

Finally, some entrepreneurs are interested in developing "human-device interfaces" (neurotechnology) that could potentially restore lost brain function. How the technology would synchronize with the brain's complex function, which is poorly understood, is a critical question.

Functional MRI and other technologies

One coma-related development that I find most worrisome is measuring the condition with tests rather than by examining a patient. Doing so can lead to overinterpretation of EEG or functional MRI — looking at brain wave activity to see "if anyone's home."

Functional MRI shows human brain activity in high resolution. On it we can see how brain regions are connected in networks and identify the regions potentially most important to an individual's recovery. It's deceptive to claim that very slow activity indicates a nonfunctional brain when someone is in a dreamless sleep and under anesthesia. We just don't know if that's the case. And some people believe that individuals with brain injuries who are unresponsive are covertly conscious — conscious but unable to tell others.

Functional MRI has been used on "locked-in" patients as well as those in presumably vegetative states to confirm that these individuals are, in fact, conscious. It's also been used to assess which regions of the brain are becoming more (or less) activated as someone begins to recover from brain injury. Generally, however, increased activity in one region that's associated with activity in another region doesn't mean that any sort of communication or direct connection is occurring between those areas. However, the regions could be critical for consciousness recovery.

Most institutions don't have protocols for using functional MRI, and the technology is expensive. One major concern is that comparisons between clinical findings and functional MRI are only valid if the examination is highly skilled and the technology is used correctly. I'm not so sure this is always the case.

Whether functional MRI adds value to a detailed, expert neurologic examination is unknown. The number of comatose patients in whom it's been studied can be counted on two hands. And estimates indicate in that 1 in 5 healthy volunteers tested, functional MRI may show no interpretable activity. And once we have the results, what do we do with them?

The science of functional MRI is fascinating. Indeed, it may eventually increase our understanding and improve treatment and decision-making for individuals with severe brain injury. But reports have often promised more than the technology can deliver (see below).

For now, I believe it best for academicians to debate, critique and synthesize data from future MRI studies that produce questionable conclusions, particularly reports that are preliminary and based on single cases — but not to share them widely with the public.

For many researchers, functional MRI offers access to the holy grail of awareness, which is understanding what happens when someone is in a coma. Does the person's mind simply go blank, or is an inner life present that the person is unable to communicate? I don't mean rare situations (for example, locked-in syndrome) in which patients can't communicate and remember being unable to do so when they've recovered. Patients coming out of a coma don't remember anything. Those who claim they do weren't comatose in the first place.

Meanwhile, technology continues to evolve, and its role in diagnosis and treatment continues to be explored. Many new technologies are still reserved for comprehensive research projects and not used in day-to-day clinical practice, where decisions based on them could produce serious consequences for an individual.

Artificial intelligence (AI) is another example of a potential future technology. But don't expect hospitals, even top-rated ones, to begin using AI for some time. How might AI one day be used? Usually, an EEG, the test that detects abnormalities in brain waves, is interpreted by experts based on what they see with their own eyes. One day, however, a "trained," computerized neural network may be just as good or better than humans at reading EEGs and using that information to predict prognosis.

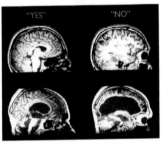

Trace of Thought Is Found in 'Vegetative' Patient

By BENEDICT CAREY

He emerged from the car accident alive but alone, there and not there: a young man whose eyes opened yet whose brain seemed shut down. For five years he lay mute and immobile beneath a diagnosis — "vegetative state" — that all but ruled out the possibility of thought, much less recovery.

But in recent months at a clinic in Liège, Belgium, the patient, now 29, showed traces of brain activity in response to commands from doctors. Now, according to a new report, he has begun to communicate: in response to simple questions, like "Do you have any brothers?," he showed distinct traces of activity on a brain imaging machine that represented either "yes" or "no."

Experts said Wednesday that the finding could alter the way some severe head injuries were diagnosed — and could raise troubling ethical questions about whether to consult severely disabled patients on their care.

The new report, posted online by The New England Journal of Medicine, does not suggest that most apparently unresponsive patients can communicate or are likely to recover. The hidden ability displayed by the young accident victim is rare, the study suggested.

Nor does the finding apply to victims of severe oxygen depletion, like Terri Schiavo, the Florida woman who became unresponsive after her heart stopped and who was taken off life support in 2005 during an explosive controversy over patients' rights.

Moreover, experts said the new test was not ready for wide use; serious technical challenges remain to be worked out.

Still, the experts agreed that the new study exposed the limits of the current bedside test for diagnosing mental state: checking whether patients' eyes can track objects, and carefully looking for any signs — eye blinks, finger twitches — in response to questions or commands.

"I'm convinced as an observer that in these few cases, the M.R.I. technique, in these researchers' hands, gives us a window into human consciousness that we have not had and that potentially adds

to the clinical exam we currently use," said Dr. James L. Bernat, a professor of neurology at Dartmouth Medical School.

In the new paper, researchers in Britain and Belgium studied 54 patients living in states of persistent unconsciousness. Of these, 23 had a diagnosis of "vegetative state," meaning they were not able to signal any response to commands or questions. (The others were termed "minimally conscious," meaning they were intermittently able to respond to commands by moving or blinking.)

In 2006, the same research

Continued on Page A20

Scans show brain activations in, above, a healthy person as he answers "yes" or "no" to a question and, below, in someone whom doctors have deemed to be in a vegetative state .

A report on functional MRI comparing findings from a healthy individual and a comatose patient. (Source: *The New York Times*. Used with permission.)

Until a multicentered trial has been carried out, however, it's too early to tell if AI can validly predict outcomes in people who are comatose.

Stem cells

Scientists have identified functional neural stem cells (NSCs) in the brains of mature mammals, and progress has been made in generating neural stem cells in lab cultures. Those two advances have raised the possibility that stem cell-based therapy could repair and regenerate the brain after trauma or a major injury.

The mechanisms of action for such a treatment are mostly hypothetical. NSCs are cells in the central nervous system with potential for self-renewal, and they can transform into different types. Adult-derived NSCs have been tested for stem cell therapy, but there are many challenges to be overcome before such therapy can be successful.

Researchers need to discover how to guide new neurons to the site of injury and ensure their long-term survival. Grafted stem cells must be compatible with the new host environment or they'll die. These challenges must be addressed in preclinical studies before stem cell-based therapies can be used in clinical practice.

Stem cells can either be injected into the arteries leading to the brain or directly implanted into the brain with a neurosurgical probe. The likelihood of success with treatment with NSCs will depend on how soon after an acute brain injury a patient receives them.

For example, in an animal study, administration of NSCs 3 to 24 hours after a stroke reduced death of brain cells by 50%. If the cells are administered days or weeks after the injury, how do researchers know if the improvements are related to treatment with the NSCs or simply part of the typical healing process?

In animal studies, stem cell treatment has restored injured tissues, but its use is still experimental. In theory, the treatment might be more successful in adolescents than in adults because younger brains are better able to regenerate lost neurons.

Areas of concern include a lack of data showing that stem cell transplantation provides meaningful benefits for humans. Data from preclinical (animal) studies showing that stem cells protect neurons in the brain shouldn't be misinterpreted as evidence that the treatment would be effective in humans. The bottom line is it's just too soon to even consider such a therapy for acute brain injury.

Brain transplantation

In the 1960s, brain transplants were performed on monkeys, but the experiments went nowhere. This piece of medical history is a cautionary tale and an egregious aberration. The data gained didn't pave the way for transplantation, but it vividly demonstrated how rapidly a brain declines following separation from a body. The experiments showed that a brain simply can't tolerate being without blood for the time it takes to remove it from the donor and reattach it to major vessels in the recipient.

Recently, the topic of brain transplantation came up again in relation to experiments in mice and a new protocol described in the media and even in medical literature. Clearly, there's still a misunderstanding about whether a brain can be transplanted into an otherwise healthy body.

Actually, the opposite seems more likely, although it's more in the realm of a horror movie than medical science. The idea is that a full-body transplant could potentially benefit a patient who has a fatal condition, such as a hereditary muscle disease that makes the body dysfunctional but leaves the brain intact. The donor would have to be a young, brain-dead individual with healthy organs of the same height, matched for immunotype, and screened for any systemic disorder. The aim would be to remove the head from the recipient and detach the body from the donor and, ultimately, transplant the recipient's head onto the healthy donor body.

Head transplantation is impossible. Recently, an attempt at fusing the two in a human model (actually, two recently deceased donors) was performed. The scientific community greeted news of this experiment with major skepticism because even attempting the procedure on deceased donors raises so many surgical, ethical and psychosocial issues.

The procedure should logically be called a "body transplant," but I don't believe for a minute that anyone has the knowledge needed to connect the head from one person to the body of another person.

AND FINALLY

Many different acute and chronic diseases and conditions can cause a coma. So, it's fruitless to think that one therapy could help every individual who is comatose. Scientists wouldn't do research on interventions for pain without knowing what led to the discomfort, and the same is true for coma.

Much of the research on new therapies for comatose patients isn't disease-specific, so why do we think these studies will result in something that will change the condition for all patients?

Rather than searching for a single therapy, research on treatments for acute coma that produces awakening and good brain function must proceed differently.

Outcomes for patients will improve if we are able to achieve the following measures of care:
1. Reduce early complications, such as increased brain pressure, shock and poor oxygenation
2. Recognize that some individuals will get worse quickly unless we take preventive steps

3. Include a neurosurgeon on the care team, because the timing of surgery matters
4. Get the little things right and avoid treatments that can harm patients
5. Standardize major interventions rather than taking a scattershot approach, with one neurorehabilitation center doing one thing while the another does something else

Greater access to a neurorehabilitation center may improve the chances of survival in a patient in a prolonged coma. This may be partly due to the use of aggressive preventive measures, such as physical therapy, and prompt, aggressive treatment of inevitable medical complications. Drug therapy to stimulate brain function is prioritized in neurorehabilitation centers, but its benefit remains questionable at best. Availability remains a major issue.

Care priorities based on sound evidence and proof also are essential, as is palliative care. The worst thing that physicians can do is just give something new "a try," without anticipating possible consequences.

Ideally, we all should be aware of the facts in order to discern what might be helpful and what might not. Trying everything isn't always the wisest plan, and families need to be warned that some therapies and interventions lack a scientific basis and are contrived and even coercive.

Additionally, some interventions are prohibitively expensive and could potentially bankrupt families. It's a crucial task for physicians to judge these claims on their merits because so much is at stake.

But none of this will make much difference if we don't connect with families — next of kin and close family members — to reach the right decisions for their loved ones.

Notes

Frequently asked questions

Chances are, you've left a hospital room or conference forgetting to ask an important question. You may have been unsure what to ask, or perhaps you were uneasy bringing up a certain topic. It happens all the time.

I understand that families often feel overwhelmed when meeting with the team that's taking care of their loved ones, particularly if many staff members are present. Families may view such meetings as coming to terms with "the writing on the wall." This isn't always the case. Doctors use family conferences to share what they know, anticipate loved ones' questions and concerns, and, above all, provide transparency. During these meetings, family members may be at a loss for words or leave the meeting with feelings of unresolved business.

In this section, I've compiled a list of 25 questions I've been asked. I hope the answers can help families better understand a loved one's condition. I've also included a checklist of topics that might improve communication and enable everyone involved to get on the same page. Not all questions will apply to every family's situation, and some have to do with very specific circumstances.

1 **Can someone who's comatose feel pain? How about someone who seems to have some awareness?**

Brain injury often affects the areas of the brain that connect feeling and affection with pain receptors. Some individuals who are comatose can only feel pain after regaining some degree of awareness. If a patient is showing signs of improvement, a physician may recommend early pain treatment. When doctors are uncertain as to the pain sensations felt by someone who's minimally conscious, we assume that the individual's capacity for pain is close to normal. So, we'll treat the pain because that's likely to do less harm than ignoring it. Similarly, providing an individual with rest and calm may improve overall well-being. However, it's very questionable to treat a deeply comatose patient for pain when the person undergoes a medical or surgical procedure known to cause physical pain because there simply is no awareness.

2 Why are food and liquids not given to someone receiving palliative care? Won't the person get hungry or thirsty?

Neither hunger nor thirst registers in patients who are comatose or who have a devastating brain injury. Many patients who've recovered some level of consciousness also may refuse to eat or drink even when it's encouraged. Their minds have changed to such a degree that hunger and thirst are secondary considerations. They're often more preoccupied with discomfort.

In someone with a devastating brain injury, after withdrawal of nutrition, fluids and medication, death is peaceful. However, decisions are far more difficult if a patient has had a feeding tube for years. Suddenly removing the tube seems intuitively cruel, and family members may disagree about removing it. These disagreements may become extreme and uncompromising and can even end up in court cases.

This happened with Terri Schiavo. Several physicians said she was very much awake and may experience normal sensations of hunger and thirst, but they based it on edited videos of Schiavo and never examined her. Many experts in neurology were unconvinced because there was no other evidence that Schiavo was conscious. The situation quickly became a political and media circus, and the courts ultimately granted Michael Schiavo's request that his wife's feeding tube be removed.

In my experience, I have often been able to resolve disagreements by taking the time to explain in detail why removing a feeding tube isn't inhumane and sometimes is the right thing to do given the previously stated wishes of the patient.

3 We keep hearing the term medically induced coma. Could you explain it?

It's unusual for a patient to be placed in a medically induced coma. What we mean by that is a patient is purposefully placed in a deep state of unconsciousness with the use of strong sedative medications.

This may be done after cardiac arrest, when a patient's body temperature is lowered to 32 or 36 C in an attempt to slow brain metabolism and help protect the brain. During cooling, sedative medications are used so that the patient is unaware of the temperature drop and doesn't shiver. Sometimes, coma is medically induced so that a mechanical ventilator can provide breaths without the patient fighting the ventilator.

Once sedative drugs are withdrawn, most patients awaken quickly and do well. Sometimes, awakening may take many days because the critical illness that brought the person to the hospital is affecting other organs, such as the kidneys and liver, and it's taking longer to clear the medications from the body. It's also possible that a patient may remain unconscious after medication withdrawal due to injuries.

4 **We've heard that an MRI can tell us if our loved one is "in there." Is that true?**

A worrisome practice on the horizon is measuring coma with tests rather than through physical examination. This may lead to overinterpretation of EEG or functional MRI results — that is, looking at a patient's test results to "see if anyone's home." There's too much we don't know and can't prove, and it's deceptive to claim that very slow activity on EEG indicates a nonfunctioning cerebral cortex when actually the person is in a dreamless sleep and under anesthesia. Conversely, the claim is often made that unresponsive patients with brain injuries are covertly conscious — that is, conscious but they don't look it — but we need to avoid making hard claims here.

Functional MRI shows different tasks happening in different areas of the brain, even in seemingly unconscious patients. But just because we're able to see some activity doesn't necessarily prove there is conscious comprehension in a person who's comatose.

5 **We've heard that tests for street drugs and other substances that are toxic aren't reliable. Is that true?**

Toxicology screening is useful, but physicians understand it has major limitations. It's simply not possible to screen for every drug, and many drugs can't be detected in blood or urine. Also, each hospital laboratory may do toxicology screening differently. Testing for barbiturates, acetaminophen, alcohol, salicylates and tricyclic antidepressants is common, and many drugs fall into one of these categories. However, what family members can tell us about a patient, such as whether the person has struggled with addiction, is often more important than what we can learn from a test.

6 **Can you tell from a CT scan whether bleeding in the brain has stopped?**

It's possible after viewing a series of images but generally not from a single scan. Many times, bleeding in the brain increases in the first hours after a patient has been injured. That's certainly true if the individual has been given medication to prevent clotting but not so much with aspirin. With trauma, doctors might see very little bleeding on the first scan and a lot more on the second one. Bruises (contusions) can gradually "blossom," and later scans may show larger areas of bleeding or bleeding in new places.

7 Our loved one always said, "I'd rather be dead than disabled." How do we make decisions knowing what he said?

Key considerations here are the extent of the disability and your loved one's willingness or ability to adapt. Profound depression and even thoughts of suicide are common in people who are newly disabled after an injury or disease. Eventually, however, some individuals adapt to their new situation, rethink their attitudes toward the disability, and decide to try to make the most of their limited function. Sometimes, people become so driven by adversity that they achieve more than ever before. Human beings can adapt to almost any situation, finding satisfaction in the smaller things they can achieve and deriving happiness from their relationships with family and friends.

Undoubtedly, however, some illnesses and impairments are extremely difficult for many individuals to endure. It's the physician's task to share the extent of the disability and explain in detail what living with it will mean. It's not expected that most people will adapt to a state in which they are speechless, bedridden, fed by tubes, and have severe contractures of the limbs. However, some patients have displayed remarkable abilities to overcome and adapt to a major injury.

8 Our loved one didn't have an advance directive, and he never talked about his wishes. How do we make decisions about worst-case scenarios?

Many people never get around to preparing an advance directive or living will, or they're reluctant to do so. Most young people don't expect to die of a major head injury or stroke. When a tragedy like that happens, the person's family must somehow come to a firm decision about how their loved one would have dealt with the situation.

It's not always possible to know how someone might respond to a disability, but few people would want a life completely devoid of pleasure. I've seen some patients accept their new disability graciously, while others respond with frustration and anger. Individuals who are initially accepting may later become uncontrollable, unreasonable, and even abusive to themselves or others. Just because someone had a lovely personality doesn't guarantee the person will retain it after a major brain injury. Even a formerly kind person can become mean and difficult, but the opposite never occurs. A common misconception is that a loved one can simply start over again and relearn what's been lost. Rehabilitation is about learning to make adjustments.

When family members are struggling to make decisions for a loved one who didn't have a living will, I suggest that they think about how their loved one responded previously to major frustrations, hospitalizations or major health issues that caused significant limitations. Memories of those times may indicate which decision to make. I also recommend having lengthy, prolonged discussions with a physician. Such discussions almost always lead to a satisfactory resolution.

9 Is it OK to ask what a physician would do for a family member in a similar situation?

I'm asked questions similar to this all of the time. It's a question that harkens back to a time when physicians had or were given much more autonomy in making decisions about how to proceed with care. Today, we practice shared decision-making with patients and families.

Even with shared decision-making, it's still important that physicians be allowed to give family members an honest assessment of how they feel about what's happening and what will happen in the future. Family members should be reassured that they have the benefit of a physician's seniority and experience as well as the physician's personal opinion.

What physicians would do for their own family members should never be different from what they would support for a patient.

10 Which physician is responsible for our loved one, and who else is on the health care team?

Families shouldn't have to ask this question. They should be told right away who the attending physician is and who else is caring for their loved one and their roles. That significantly improves trust and understanding. I always tell families clearly who's on the team. They need to know who the primary physician is and who is co-primary (that is, providing the same level of care but with another expertise). Families should also be made aware of how shifts work and when to expect staff changes.

TOPICS TO DISCUSS WITH YOUR HEALTH CARE TEAM

- Comfort
- Expectations
- Surgery
- Complications
- Lifesaving measures
- Long-term care
- Insurance
- Social work

11 Can we get a second opinion?

Yes. And it's often easy to get one in the hospital. That's because many physicians in a hospital will have already reviewed all or part of a patient's case. For example, the neuroradiologist who reviewed a patient's brain scans may have asked another neuroradiologist to review them as well. Family members may not be aware of such consultations.

No physician with any scruples would balk at a family's request for a second opinion. It will be useful if the person providing the second opinion:

- Is senior level, knowledgeable and experienced about the condition and has never taken care of the individual
- Has the skills to fully evaluate the patient independently and examines him or her under the best circumstances
- Reaches a conclusion, discusses the findings with the attending physician, and resolves differences, if possible
- Acknowledges the possibility that there may be a different interpretation of the patient's situation
- Discusses the findings with family members and documents them

The problem with second opinions can be conformity bias. That is the desire to agree with the strongest, most convincing opinion and to trust the judgment of others rather than your own.

12 What if I strongly disagree with someone on the health care team who's taking care of my loved one? What should I do?

Caring for a loved one who's comatose is stressful. Understandably, some family members have little patience left. Maintaining an open line of communication with your loved one's doctor while also voicing and discussing your concerns remains key and often will restore trust.

When trust between family and the health care team erodes, the relationship may turn sour. If that happens, a patient's family members can always request that a different member of the team care for their loved one. Asking for a second opinion and transferring the patient to another hospital are both options if conflicts can't be resolved.

Negligence and even medical errors do occur, but they're rarely a result of bad systems. Hospitals take issues involving patient safety very seriously. Certainly, they want to avoid risk of liability and lawsuits, but mostly they have a genuine desire to do good and avoid doing harm.

13 We're afraid that insurance won't cover our loved one's care. How do we get financial support?

Physicians understand that long-term care is extremely expensive for families. Social workers play a very important role in helping families identify forms of support for long-term care. They become involved as soon as a comatose patient is admitted to the intensive care unit, and they pursue the best benefits available through insurance or other programs and community resources.

Health insurance doesn't always cover all expenses. Long-term care insurance or Medicaid may cover some of the costs.

Some hospitals also have special funds established to assist patients who are uninsured. It's very important to meet regularly with a social worker, who can help locate programs to assist with ongoing expenses.

14 We can't afford long-term care for our loved one. How can a facility deny him what he needs?

There's just no easy way to put this. Denying care based on a family's inability to pay for it is immoral. Denying care because someone is underinsured is, too. On the other hand, the high cost of caring for people who are terminally ill and have devastating, neurologic conditions is problematic. Health care systems are imperfect.

The challenges of access to medical care and the cost of medical care in the United States are beyond the scope of this book, and even experts on the subject have trouble grappling with it. In most countries, socioeconomic factors are the main drivers of health, not the health care system itself. Poverty plays a crucial role. In countries with a tax-financed universal health care system ("socialized medicine"), mortality remains high among low-income patients with certain diseases. Gaps in life expectancy by income level are substantial and continue to increase in Norway and the United Kingdom, even though they have near-universal health care and less income inequality than in the United States. These problems can't

be fixed overnight, and they may never be solved.

What I do know is that most major medical institutions have ways to help families overwhelmed by the cost of care for a loved one. Social workers have experience in finding ways for families to avoid financial disaster. Charity care and other options are available for uninsured patients. One of my patients who recovered from a coma told me that his only worry was how to cope with all the medical bills. It shouldn't be that way. Even in economically good times, many families still can't cope with the financial strain of chronic illness in a loved one.

15 How soon after all treatment is stopped will our loved one die? Should we tell family members who live far away to come right away?

This is a common question, but unfortunately, it's difficult to answer with certainty. If a patient is barely breathing on a ventilator, the heart will stop quickly after the machine is removed. But death may take much longer if the person is breathing well on a ventilator. Once off a ventilator, someone who is comatose may breathe comfortably at first, superficially for several days, and die in 7 to 10 days. Before a patient transitions to full comfort care, we make sure all his or her loved ones have had the opportunity to say goodbye. It's common to wait until everyone who wants to be present has come, even if it takes a few days' travel for some family members. No one should die alone, even individuals who are unconscious.

16 Has a patient who was expected to die ever surprised you and gotten better when the ventilator was removed?

No. Patients with devastating neurologic illnesses don't improve after a ventilator is removed. That's not to say that physicians don't make mistakes. There are cases of patients in hospices improving, but a major change is very unlikely. What usually happens after a comatose individual's tubes and lines are removed is a gradual and peaceful death.

17 Do you ever worry that you might be wrong about a patient who is comatose?

Physicians aren't all-knowing, and we're constantly called upon to predict what's going to happen to our patients. As human beings, we're humbled when we're proven wrong, whether we expected a poor outcome and a patient recovers or the opposite happens. Some physicians think it's inappropriate to discuss outcome at all. But in my experience, medical care can only function if physicians set goals and make judgments.

We have an obligation to inform family members. Without putting a number on it, we should always ask ourselves, "What are the odds?" Moreover, physicians should be reluctant doomsayers, although it's our duty to be honest with families even when the information we must share about their loved one is truly bad.

18 Is there any new device that can help our loved one? We've heard about brain stimulators.

This is a true conundrum. It's easy to fixate on the grandiose possibilities of modern technology without considering whether it's feasible or potentially harmful. The real mantra for technology should be, "It's not what you could do with it; it's whether you should do it." We could do quite a lot. We could give patients experimental drugs or implant brain stimulators. But should we do it?

Use of such technology is a gamble. Will advances in neuroscience help patients who would otherwise be forgotten and marginalized? Or will they create false hope and, in the end, terrible emotional and financial costs? We must move very cautiously with any new intervention, particularly if we don't know whether it could cause harm. Psychosurgery with implantation of electrodes in the brain and ultrasound have been very successful for patients with certain types of Parkinson's disease and familial tremors, for instance. But they haven't worked in treating disorders of consciousness.

The greatest progress after traumatic brain injury generally occurs in patients with good mental function who can be trained to use a device. Most recently, neural prostheses activated by brain implants have allowed moderately paralyzed people to open and close their hands. Some devices also are able to translate brain activity to speech. Unquestionably, this is an exciting area.

19 Will I have regrets later about the decisions I've made for my loved one?

In all the years I've been practicing, I can only recall one time that a family member expressed regret about not doing more for a loved one who was comatose. Surveys of spouses and children of comatose patients show that they have very little regret about their decisions. Challenges typically arise when family members feel that their own goals and values differ from those of the patient. In these situations, we focus on shared decision-making and emphasize the concept of self-determination and the need to honor an individual's wishes if they're known.

20 I've heard that brain death doesn't mean that a person is really dead. Is that true?

Some scholars, bioethicists and theologians do question the concept of brain death. However, it's been recognized in clinical practice around the world for nearly half a century. No experts in

neurology and neurosurgery have questioned the definition of brain death since it was first described. Most of them agree that death of the brain is sufficient to declare an individual dead.

In my estimation, people who criticize brain death as a concept are making a negative judgment about the abilities of physicians to determine whether a neurologic injury is irreversible. They may also insinuate that medical professionals involved in making such decisions lack respect for a patient's life.

Neurologists and other physicians caring for individuals in a coma have a clear definition of death. The presence and uniformity of laws defining death, including brain death, have been adopted and are widely accepted. Any other position that falls outside the scope of conventional thinking could greatly compromise the integrity of medical professionals. Accommodating a family's request to continue support in a patient who is declared dead by neurologic criteria raises tremendous concerns of justice and fairness and could establish a troubling precedent for the future.

In the practice of medicine, certain signs suffice for a diagnosis; in the practice of philosophy, none is definitive. Today, major Western religions support organ and tissue donation. A few Judaic and Christian scholars take issue with brain death and demand a vitalist approach. However, religious affiliation generally is not an overriding obstacle for most people when confronted with a loved one who is brain-dead and asked about organ donation. In some parts of the world, the role of faith in such decisions is more apparent.

If family members have religious or cultural objections to declaring a loved one brain-dead, it's important that they speak with their own religious leaders. In my experience, clergy can be very helpful in clarifying the meaning of brain death and the process of organ donation.

21 My spouse is brain-dead. We were planning to have a child. Can his sperm be removed so I can do in vitro fertilization?

I have great sympathy for the partners of patients who are comatose who want to harvest their partner's mature germ cells (gametes) to create a family. The practice is controversial and presents logistical problems. The American Society for Reproductive Medicine Ethics Committee has stated that "a spouse's request that sperm or ova be obtained terminally or soon after death without the prior consent or known wishes of the deceased spouse need not be honored."

Hospital policies may also specifically require an advance directive, written or verbal, with evidence of implied consent from the patient. Without written consent, some argue, it's difficult to know what the deceased would have wanted. But such a legal document is unlikely to exist, because, frankly, who would think to prepare it? A spouse's request may still be carefully considered in some situations,

such as if the couple was already trying to conceive through artificial insemination.

In the absence of a written directive, physicians aren't obligated to comply with a request from a surviving spouse or partner to obtain a deceased patient's gametes.

There's no information on the success of such retrieval procedures, particularly in patients who are brain-dead. And sperm from critically ill patients may be of poor quality. In addition, most insurance plans won't cover the high costs involved in these fertility-related procedures.

22 Is our loved one too old to be a donor?

Age isn't a criterion for organ donation. At the time of an individual's death, the transplant team determines if organ donation is a possibility. The oldest donor to date was age 93. Even a person with medical conditions can be an eye and tissue donor.

23 I know someone who's been waiting a long time for an organ transplant. Can that person get my loved one's organs?

In the United States, it's legal for families who agree to organ donation to ask that the organs be given to family members or friends. They can also choose which organs to donate. Any person in need of an organ transplant can receive it as a gift from a family member. Most commonly, this practice involves donation by living donors, but it can also apply to brain-dead donors.

To eliminate any possible conflict of interest, it's important for physicians to ensure that the determination of brain death is fully separated from any discussion about organ donation. If family members agree to a directed donation, the organ-procurement agency will attempt to honor that wish. Directing a gift, however, is only the first decision in the process of matching the donor with the recipient, and it may not work if the donor and the recipient are incompatible.

However, family members can't put other restrictions on organ donation, such as refusing to give a liver to someone who misused alcohol or drugs. The United Network for Organ Sharing (UNOS) has carefully worded guidelines for such a situation. They say, "Donation of organs may not be made in a manner which discriminates against a person or class of persons on the basis of race, national origin, religion, gender or similar characteristic."

24 How much does organ donation cost? Do we get paid if our loved one's organs are donated?

The entire cost of organ donation is paid by the organ-procurement organization. Generally, this includes all costs from the time brain death is declared to when the donor's body is transferred to a medical examiner or funeral home. The donor's family isn't compensated. In the United States, the sale of organs is prohibited and punishable.

25 Do you have to be dead to donate organs?

Only a single kidney and a lobe of the liver can be taken from a living donor. Removing the lungs, heart or other complete organs isn't possible because it would lead to immediate death.

Some ethicists believe that organs should be removed from any patient who has no chance of survival, without waiting for death. These individuals claim — and wrongly, in my opinion — that doctors "kill all the time" by stopping life support. It can't be denied that withdrawing life-sustaining treatment eventually leads to death. However, taking the heart from a breathing, still-moving patient is a very different matter.

Moreover, where do we draw the line? No competent clinical team would be prepared to assist a person in a self-sacrificing organ donation. The idea contravenes the code of conduct of all professional medical organizations.

Suggested readings

Most of the resources in this section are from the medical literature. I've included important works on coma as well as current information about interventions for managing the condition. My goal is to give readers insight into why I said certain things in this book and how opinions about coma have been formed over the years. Some publications are specifically mentioned in the chapters, and you can find further explanation in the full references, listed here.

Some of the resources are scientific and esoteric, and the concepts may be difficult to understand. Therefore, the listings here were chosen based on readability and relevance. Many books have been written about the experience of having a loved one with a brain injury, some of them describing prolonged coma.

Among the authors are journalists, science writers and families telling their own stories. Their experiences and interpretations fill the spectrum from very good to very bad.

Guide to the Comatose Patient concentrates on the interactions of family members and health care teams in the real world and "in the trenches." In the last decade, new data has emerged in academic literature about the importance of family-physician relationships. Those of us in the medical profession study this closely so that it can guide us in providing better care to our patients. Personally, I believe it's preferable to rely on carefully vetted medical literature to connect the dots rather than being guided only by personal opinions and experiences.

CHAPTER 1

A statement from a multidisciplinary group of rehabilitation physicians and neurology researchers. A comprehensive summary of types of prolonged coma and neurorehabilitation options (and limitations).

Giacino JT, et al. Comprehensive systematic review update summary: Disorders of consciousness — Report of the Guideline Development, Dissemination, and Implementation Subcommittee of the American Academy of Neurology. *Neurology.* 2018;91:461.

The first detailed descriptions of vegetative state and a follow-up assessment years later. The book is a classic work on vegetative state by the late neurosurgeon Brian Jennett and a cumulation of his life's work. His views on ethical and legal dilemmas were prescient.

Jennett B, Plum F. Persistent vegetative state after brain damage. A syndrome in search of a name. *Lancet.* 1972;1:734. Jennett B. The vegetative state. *Journal of Neurology, Neurosurgery and Psychiatry.* 2002; 73:355. Jennett B. The Vegetative State. Medical Facts, Ethical and Legal Dilemmas. Cambridge University Press; 2002.

A summary of the differences between minimally conscious state and vegetative state and how they can look alike.

Wijdicks EF. Minimally conscious state versus persistent vegetative state: The case of Terri (Wallis) versus Terri (Schiavo). *Mayo Clinic Proceedings.* 2006;81:1155.

A detailed account of a locked-in syndrome.

Laureys S, et al. The locked-in syndrome: what is it like to be conscious but paralyzed and voiceless? *Progress in Brain Research.* 2005;150:495.

CHAPTER 2

A book summarizing at least 100 potential causes of coma described in detail.

Wijdicks EFM. The Comatose Patient. 2nd edition. Oxford University Press; 2016.

An early study depicting a rapid rise in opioid cases. Currently nearly 50,000 Americans die of an opioid-related overdose, more than 130 lives each day.

Hasegawa K, et al. Epidemiology of emergency department visits for opioid overdose: a population-based study. *Mayo Clinic Proceedings.* 2014;89:462.

CHAPTER 3

An account of what neurologists often do when they make a diagnosis and initiate treatment.

Wijdicks EF. The bare essentials: Coma. *Practical Neurology.* 2010;10:51.

A witty but true explanation why the ABCs in resuscitation often isn't enough.

Guly HR. ABCDEs. *Emergency Medicine Journal.* 2003;20:358.

A discussion of the pathophysiology and cause of coma; practical clinical aspects of coma; and how to obtain correct historical information, perform a thorough physical examination, order appropriate testing and imaging studies, and provide appropriate treatment.

> Traub SJ, et al. Initial diagnosis and management of coma. *Emergency Medicine Clinics North America.* 2016;34:777.

redesign. *Annals of the American Thoracic Society.* 2020;17:221.

A review of critically ill patients with COVID-19 in the intensive care unit who take much longer to awaken than normally expected.

> Edlow BL, et al. Delayed reemergence of consciousness in survivors of severe COVID-19. *Neurocritical Care.* 2020;33:627.

CHAPTER 4

A cohort of more than 15,000 patients with traumatic brain injury demonstrating about 40% of patients admitted to rehabilitation centers with a disorder of consciousness achieved nearly full independence.

> Kowalski RG, et al. Recovery of consciousness and functional outcome in moderate and severe traumatic brain injury. *JAMA Neurology.* 2021;78:548.

A critical assessment of prediction models and their serious limitations. The potential negative consequences of wrong estimates of severity are detailed.

> Tenovuo O, et al. Assessing the severity of traumatic brain injury — Time for a change? *Journal of Clinical Medicine.* 2021;10:148.

An article on issues encountered after leaving the ICU and the priorities of patients soon to be discharged to go home.

> Scheunemann L et al. Post-intensive care unit care: A qualitative analysis of patient priorities and implications for

CHAPTER 5

A classic article on how certain medical language suggests confidence, but is, in fact, a lot of guesswork.

> Rappeport JR. Reasonable medical certainty. *Bulletin of the American Academy of Psychiatry and Law.* 1985;13:5.

A recent study on ways to improve communication regarding patient goals. Stages outlined include sharing knowledge, clarifying goals of care and negotiating treatment options.

> Lu E, et al. A "three stage protocol" for serious illness conversations: Reframing communication in real time. *Mayo Clinic Proceedings.* 2020;95:1589.

Insight into what worries family members, including the ability to predict patient outcome with accuracy.

> Hwang DY, et al. Concerns of surrogate decision makers for patients with acute brain injury: A US population survey. *Neurology.* 2020;94:e2054.

A look at how family members interpret and perceive prognostic data in response to how it's presented.

Chapman AR, et al. The effect of prognostic data presentation format on perceived risk among surrogate decision makers of critically ill patients: A randomized comparative trial. *Journal of Critical Care*. 2015;30:231.

CHAPTER 6

A study on racial disparities in end-of-life care and identifying groups with different approaches.

Orlovic M, et al. Racial and ethnic differences in end-of-life care in the United States: Evidence from the Health and Retirement Study (HRS). *SSM-Population Health*. 2019;7:100331.

A major study of patients with a traumatic brain injury who are comatose, identifying social and race factors that influence the decision to withdraw support.

Williamson T, et al. Withdrawal of life-supporting treatment in severe traumatic brain injury. *JAMA Surgery*. 2020;155:723.

A look at anxieties experienced by physicians when making end-of-life decisions.

Turgeon AF, et al. Factors influencing decisions by critical care physicians to withdraw life-sustaining treatments in critically ill adult patients with severe traumatic brain injury. *Canadian Medical Association Journal*. 2019;191:E652.

The role of families in the intensive care unit, serving as both facilitators and historians for the patient.

McAdam JL, et al. Unrecognized contributions of families in the intensive care unit. *Intensive Care Medicine*. 2008;34:1097.

Stress reactions experienced by family members after a loved one is discharged from the intensive care unit or dies.

Azoulay E, et al. Risk of post-traumatic stress symptoms in family members of intensive care unit patients. *American Journal of Respiratory Critical Care Medicine*. 2005;171:987.

A review of important factors in surrogate decision-making and surrogate-clinician communication.

Vig E, et al. Surviving surrogate decision-making: What helps and hampers the experience of making medical decisions for others. *Journal of General Internal Medicine*. 2007;22:1274.

A review of how physicians use numbers and how surrogates' understanding of numbers may affect goals-of-care decisions.

Leiter N, et al. Numeracy and interpretation of prognostic estimates in intracerebral hemorrhage among surrogate decision makers in the neurologic ICU. *Critical Care Medicine*. 2018;46:264.

CHAPTER 7

Important observations on family experiences concerning organ donation.

Kerstis B, et al. When life ceases: Relatives' experiences when a family member is confirmed brain dead and becomes a potential organ donor — A literature review. *Sage Open Nursing.* 2020;6:2377960820922031.

A summary of ethnic, religious and bioethical perspectives of organ donation.

Da Silva IRF, et al. Worldwide barriers to organ donation. *JAMA.* 2015;72:112.

A predictor of cardiac death after ventilator removal resulting in successful organ donation.

Rabinstein AA, et al. Prediction of potential for organ donation after cardiac death in patients in neurocritical state: A prospective observational study. *The Lancet Neurology.* 2012;11:414.

A landmark study on grief and navigating organ donation.

Kentish-Barnes N, et al. Grief symptoms in relatives who experienced organ donation requests in the ICU. *American Journal of Respiratory and Critical Care Medicine.* 2018;198:751.

An extension of a previous study offering important new insights into the difficulties of organ donation when the patient's wishes are unknown.

Kentish-Barnes N, et al. Being nonvinced and taking responsibility: A qualitative study of family members' experience of organ donation decision and bereave-ment after brain death. *Critical Care Medicine.* 2019;47:526.

A large-scale review on brain death and organ donation. Clinical determination, tests, precautions and pitfalls, and legal, ethical and religious topics are discussed.

Wijdicks EFM. Brain Death. 3rd ed. Oxford University Press; 2017.

CHAPTER 8

The first comprehensive paper on living wills with an attempt to put some stops on escalation of care.

Kutner L. Due process of euthanasia: The living will, a proposal. *Indiana Law Journal.* 1969;44:539.

The first article on limiting care in hospital patients and a landmark discussion on compassionate care.

Rabkin MT, et al. Orders not to resuscitate. *New England Journal of Medicine.* 1976;295:364.

One of the first papers suggesting physicians may be do harm by providing ongoing care to a vulnerable patient in coma.

Cassem NH. Confronting the decision to let death come. *Critical Care Medicine* 1974; 2(3):113-117.

Survey results of donor families on their experiences with organ and tissue donation.

Savaria DT, et al. Donor family surveys provide useful information for organ procurement. *Transplantation Proceedings.* 1990;22:316.

A landmark paper on the need to provide care when there is no hope. This influential paper preceded the author's work on the Harvard committee to define brain death.

Beecher HK. After the "definition of irreversible coma." *New England Journal of Medicine*. 1969;281:1070.

An argument to allow organ donation without documentation of death. The argument remains highly controversial.

Truog RD, et al. The dead donor rule and organ transplantation. *New England Journal of Medicine*. 2008;359:674.

A discussion of end-of-life care as it relates to care for the patient, using appropriate sedation.

Billings JA. Humane terminal extubation reconsidered: The role for preemptive analgesia and sedation. *Critical Care Medicine*. 2012;40:625.

A review of how physicians might approach conversations with family members.

Truog RD, et al. Recommendations for end-of-life care in the intensive care unit: The Ethics Committee of the Society of Critical Care Medicine. *Critical Care Medicine*. 2001;29:2332.

How escalation and de-escalation of intensive care occurs and who's involved.

Brody H, et al. Withdrawing intensive life-sustaining treatment — Recommendations for compassionate clinical management. *New England Journal of Medicine*. 1997;336:652.

Involving family members in early decision-making after a brain hemorrhage.

Sahgal S, et al. Surrogate satisfaction with decision making after intracerebral hemorrhage. *Neurocritical Care*. 2021;34:193.

An internist's view as to the role of spirituality in medicine.

Matthews DA, et al. The Faith Factor: Proof of the healing power of prayer. *Penguin Books*; 1999.

The meaning of the term *Hail Mary* and how the term can be misunderstood.

Nash IS. Hail Mary. *JAMA Neurology*. 2020;77:159.

CHAPTER 9

The correlation between fewer formal family meetings and family dissatisfaction with neuro-ICU shared decision-making.

Weber U, et al. Predictors of family dissatisfaction with support during neurocritical care shared decision-making. *Neurocritical Care*. 2021;35:714.

The effect of family interventions in the ICU and staff training to improve communication on surrogates' long-term psychological distress.

White DB, et al. A randomized trial of a family-support intervention in intensive care units. *New England Journal of Medicine*. 2018;378:2365.

The effect of intensive psychosocial support for families as it relates to the duration of intensive treatment before the patient's death.

Curtis JR, et al. Randomized trial of communication facilitators to reduce family distress and intensity of end-of-life care. *American Journal of Respiratory and Critical Care Medicine.* 2016;193:154.

An overview of issues involved in making decisions for a loved one.
Wendler D, Rid A. Systematic review: The effect on surrogates of making treatment decisions for others. *Annals of Internal Medicine.* 2011;154:336.

How relationships can turn sour and the lessons learned.
Kiesewetter I, et al. Patients' perception of types of errors in palliative care — Results from a qualitative interview study. *BMC Palliative Care.* 2016;15:75.

Insights into personal perspectives and how certain interactions can lead to decisions.
Wijdicks EFM, et al. The family conference: End-of-life guidelines at work for comatose patients. *Neurology.* 2007;68:1092.

The vital role of nursing staff in discussions of care.
Lamas D. Nurse-led communication in the intensive care unit. *New England Journal of Medicine.* 2018; 378:2431.

CHAPTER 10

A review from the Cochrane Center on sensory stimulation involving patients with acute coma or prolonged coma.
Lombardi F, et al. Sensory stimulation of brain-injured individuals in coma or vegetative state: Results of a Cochrane systematic review. *Clinical Rehabilitation.* 2002;16:464.

A 20-year prospective, uncontrolled and nonrandomized observational study on the effect of spinal column stimulation on patients in persistent vegetative states.
Kanno T, et al. Dorsal column stimulation in persistent vegetative states. *Neuromodulation.* 2009;12:33.

An overview on the efficacy of various neuromodulatory therapies.
Xia X, et al. Current status of neuro-modulatory therapies for disorders of consciousness. *Neuroscience Bulletin.* 2018;34:615.

Family responses to portrayals of unconsciousness in the media.
Samuel G , et al. Reporting consciousness in coma: Media framing of neuro-scientific research, hope, and the response of families with relatives in vegetative and minimally conscious states. *Journalism, Media, and Cultural Studies Journal.* 2013;3:10244.

Interesting questions addressing expectations of health care and the functioning of health care systems during the COVID-19 pandemic.
Levy B-H. The Virus in the Age of Madness. Yale University Press; 2020.

Use of the medication zolpidem after severe brain injury.

Arnts H, et al. Awakening after a sleeping pill: Restoring functional brain networks after severe brain injury. *Cortex*. 2020;132:135.

A review of an HBO documentary on coma, concluding that a selective approach failed to recognize a far more complex problem.

Wijdicks EFM. Why the new HBO documentary, 'COMA,' is disappointing. *Neurology Today*. 2007;7:28.

Viewers reactions to coma portrayed in movies.

Wijdicks EF, et al. The portrayal of coma in contemporary motion pictures. *Neurology*. 2006;66:1300.

Newspaper headlines and coma.

Wijdicks EFM, et al. Coverage of coma in headlines of US newspapers from 2001 through 2005. *Mayo Clinic Proceedings*. 2006;81:1332.

An internet study on reliability of website descriptions of brain death.

Jones AH, et al. Investigation of public perception of brain death using the internet. *Chest*. 2018;154:286.

A study on the availability of information for families concerning organ donation after cardiac arrest.

Black K, et al. What information about donation after circulatory death is available on the Internet for potential donor families? *Clinical Transplantation*. 2016;30:934.

Ongoing debate on use of MRI in determining different types of prolonged coma.

Scolding N, et al. Prolonged disorders of consciousness: a critical evaluation of the new UK guidelines. *Brain*. 2021; 144:1655.

Nearly half of the recommendations by hosts of medical talk shows are baseless, or worse, contradict evidence.

Korownyk C, et al. Televised medical talk shows — what they recommend and the evidence to support their recommendations: A prospective observational study. *BMJ*. 2014;349:g7346.

Index

decision-making
    ability to adapt and, 188
    difficulty of, 8
    organ donation and, 126–127
    regret and, 193
    shared, 155–156, 189
    worst-case scenarios and, 188
deep vein thrombosis (DVT), 64
delirious patients, 15
depression and apathy, 73, 76
dignity, 146
direct brain injury, 37–41
donation after cardiac death (DCD), 131
do-not-resuscitate (DNR) orders,
    147–149
dorsal column stimulation, 178
drains, 59, 176
drowsy patients, 15
drug overdose
    See overdose, drug; overdose-induced
        coma
drug treatments, 174–175

E

early treatment, 55–57
electrical analogy, 20–21
electrode implantation, 177
electroencephalogram (EEG), 33, 35,
    49–51, 98, 187
emergency department, 45
emotions, 73
encephalitis, 82, 84, 96
euthanasia, 108
experimental and unproven therapies
    about, 167–168
    artificial intelligence (AI), 179–180
    brain transplantation, 180–181
    coma in the media and, 169–170
    drug treatments, 174–175
    fact versus fiction and, 168–173
    functional MRI, 178–179

levels of evidence, 173
    music therapy, 176
    neural prostheses and, 192
    sensory simulation programs,
        175–176
    stem cells, 180
    transcranial magnetic stimulation,
        177–178
extensor posturing, 24
eyes
    closure of, 23
    comatose patient and, 7, 23
    frontal lobe surgery and, 26
    locked-in syndrome and, 16
    opening of, 23, 27, 70
    seizures and, 61
    tracking with, 28–29, 30
    vegetative state and, 7, 27

F

families and family members
    acceptance and, 100
    care of, 160–161
    communication and, 8, 154–155, 162,
        163–164
    concerns expressed by, 160
    conversations with organ-procurement
        coordinators and, 162
    differences of opinion and, 160
    expectations and, 100
    final decisions and, 102
    life support withdrawal and, 124
    meeting location and, 161–163
    poor outcomes and, 100–102
    predicting outcomes and, 102
    quality of life and, 141
family conferences
    about, 162
    communication in, 163–164
    conflicts in, 164–165
    facts and the truth and, 164

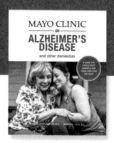
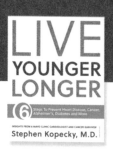
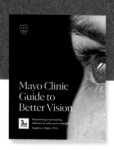
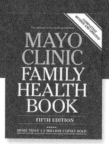
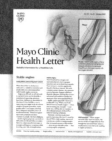